ONE ROOT, MANY RISKS

Your Roadmap to Outsmarting Cancer, Cardiovascular Disease & Memory Loss

A Prevention Playbook to Slash Your Risk Starting Today

Gabriel Gavrilescu, MD

One Root, Many Risks: Your Roadmap to Outsmarting Cancer, Cardiovascular Disease & Memory Loss

Copyright © 2025 Gavrimed LLC
Written by Gabriel Gavrilescu

All rights reserved. No part of this publication may be reproduced, stored in a retrieval system, or transmitted in any form or by any means-electronic, mechanical, photocopying, recording, or otherwise-without the prior written permission of Gavrimed LLC, except in the case of brief quotations embodied in critical articles or reviews.

Back Cover Photo: Luigi Modesti | photobyluigi.com

ISBN Paperback: 979-8-89576-135-9

Publisher: Gavrimed LLC, Fort Lauderdale, FL, USA

Published by:

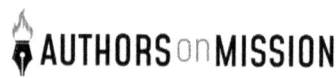

Medical disclaimer: The information in this book is provided for educational purposes only and is not a substitute for professional medical advice. Always consult your physician or other qualified healthcare provider with any questions you may have regarding a medical condition or treatment.

To Adri- my partner in every sense, my first reader and sharp editor, for your steady encouragement on this project and throughout my whole career. I couldn't have done it without you.

To Mom and Dad- for laying the foundation.

Table of Contents

Introduction 9
How to Read This Book 11
A Bit About Me 14
Chapter 1: Longevity 16
    Defining Longevity 16
    Biological Fundamentals of Longevity 16
    Evolution of Longevity: Trends Over Time 17
    Key Historical Milestones in Longevity Trends 18
    Longevity in the U.S. vs. the Rest of the World 19
    Key Factors Behind Differences in Longevity 19
    The Role of Social Determinants of Health in Longevity 19
    Future Trends in Longevity 21
    The Century with the Most Rapid Increase in Longevity 22
    Conclusion 22
Chapter 2: Mortality 23
    What the Numbers Say 23
    A Century of Change 25
    What Drives Modern Mortality? 25
    A Global Perspective 27
    The Power of Prevention 28
Chapter 3: Drivers of Risk 29
    Sugar (Glucose) 29
    Cholesterol 31
    Blood Pressure 35
    Weight 36
Chapter 4: How the Damage is Done 41
    Heart Attack / Stroke 41

    Diabetes 44

    Cancer 46

    Dementia 51

    The vicious circle linking all: the metabolic complex of diseases 54

Chapter 5: How the Damage Can Be Undone or Prevented:
                Diet, Exercise, Tobacco and Alcohol Avoidance 61

    Diet 61

    Exercise 77

    Tobacco: The One Risk Factor with No Upside 91

    Health Improvements Timeline After Quitting Smoking 95

    From Cigarettes to Spirits: Another Risk Worth Confronting 95

    Alcohol: Reconsidering the "Glass of Red Wine" 96

Chapter 6: How the Damage can be Undone or Prevented:
                Diabetes, Blood Pressure, and Cholesterol 99

    Weight and Insulin Resistance/Diabetes 99

    Metformin: A Foundational Tool for Metabolic Improvement 102

    Blood Pressure 104

    Cholesterol 113

Chapter 7: GLP-1 Receptor Agonists: A Revolutionary Medication 129

    How GLP-1 Receptor Agonists Work 130

    Precautions When Starting GLP-1 Receptor Agonists 142

    GLP-1 Receptor Agonists Treatment Cost 144

Chapter 8: Health Maintenance 147

    What is Health Maintenance? 147

    Screening for Cancer 149

    Immunizations 164

    Sleep 166

    Sleep Apnea – A Closer Look 168

    Primary Care Physician Role 169

    Social Connection and Its Health Power 172

    Summary 175

Chapter 9: Exploring Additional Health Claims 176
   No Magic Pill.. 176
   Supplements 178
   CT or MRI Scan of the Whole Body 182
   Blood Tests for Screening.. 184
   Cleansing, Detox, and IV Vitamins 186

Chapter 10: Do It Yourself: How to Set Your Weight Goal and
      the Diet Plan to Achieve It.. 190
   Step 1: Get a Digital Scale and Understand Your Body............ 190
   Step 2: Set a Realistic Weight Loss Goal 191
   Step 3: Calculate Your Total Daily Energy Expenditure (TDEE) 191
   Step 4: Set Your Caloric Deficit 192
   Step 5: Design Your Meal Plan 192
   Step 6: Track Intake Honestly... 193
   Step 7: Maintain (and Improve) Your Exercise Program 193
   Final Thoughts.. 194

Epilogue: The Common Thread, The Common Fix............................... 195

References 197

Gabriel Gavrilescu, M.D. is an internal medicine and geriatrics physician practicing at Cleveland Clinic Florida, in Weston and West Palm Beach.

Any opinions expressed in this book are those of the author and do not represent the views of Cleveland Clinic.

Introduction

The idea of writing this book had been on my mind for a while, but I never quite found the energy or motivation to start. However, three main factors have finally propelled me to take on this project, and I hope they will also drive me to see it through to completion.

The first reason is the overwhelming amount of information circulating about medical procedures, supplements, diets, and so-called "one-size-fits-all" solutions that claim to improve longevity, aid in weight management, reduce cardiovascular risk, and enhance overall well-being. Some of these claims are backed by credible evidence, but many, perhaps most, are not. What they do have in common is their profitability for those promoting them. In this book, I will strive to present data to support my key statements, drawing from reputable journals and vetted sources, so that readers can distinguish between scientifically supported practices and marketing-driven trends. I have no financial ties to any of the diets, exercise regimens, or medications I mention here. My only goal is to make this information available to those who are interested.

The second reason is my patients. In almost every clinic visit, I take time to discuss specific conditions, preventative measures, cardiovascular risk optimization, weight management, and cancer screening. At least one of these topics arises in most visits. Over the years, I have developed a way to summarize essential, meaningful, and actionable information in a concise format. This book is an extension of those efforts, an accessible resource for my patients and anyone else seeking clear, evidence-based guidance on maintaining their health. I understand that we all have short attention spans (myself included), so I will do my best to keep things brief, distill the most valuable insights, and avoid attempting an exhaustive review of every topic. There will undoubtedly be areas that I omit, some intentionally and others inadvertently, but future iterations of this book may expand on them.

Additionally, if there is significant interest, I plan to create a companion website to provide updates, as medical knowledge is constantly evolving. The ever-changing nature of medical research is one reason for widespread confusion; what we believe to be absolute truth today may be revised tomorrow. However, most of the principles I share here are well-established, supported by decades of practice and evidence. When I discuss more recent findings, I will make that distinction clear.

The third reason I finally found the stamina and momentum to write this book is the undeniable connection between longevity, cardiovascular health, cancer risk, memory loss, and other major health conditions. One of the book's key themes will be how addressing cardiovascular risk factors provides broad benefits across multiple areas of health. Diet, exercise, maintaining a healthy lifestyle, monitoring cholesterol and glucose levels, and minimizing toxins in our bodies can significantly impact not just heart health and longevity but also cancer risk, mental well-being, and overall quality of life.

How to Read This Book

This book is meant to empower, not overwhelm you. It's written for anyone who wants to better understand how the body works, how disease develops, and most importantly, how to take meaningful steps toward prevention. **You don't need a medical degree to follow along**. Each chapter builds on key ideas, connecting the dots between metabolic health, cancer, and memory disorders in a way that's practical, clear, and personal. You can read it front to back or skip around to the sections that matter most to you right now, whether that's learning how to lower blood pressure, understanding your cholesterol numbers, or designing your own diet plan. Whenever you see the word "calories," know that I'm referring to *kilocalories*, the unit we actually use in nutrition, even though common usage drops the "kilo." You'll also see occasional prompts to try with AI tools like ChatGPT. Don't be afraid to engage with them: they're here to help you turn knowledge into action. Most of all, this is your journey.

Take what's useful, come back as needed, and remember: **prevention is powerful, and it starts with understanding.**

▨■☐ DISCLAIMER: THIS BOOK IS NOT INDIVIDUAL MEDICAL ADVICE

Please read before continuing

This book is for **educational purposes only**. It is **not a substitute for professional medical care**, diagnosis, or treatment.

🧠 The information here is intended to help you better understand your health risks, debunk common myths, and guide more productive, informed discussions with your physician.

🩺 Your health decisions, about medications, screenings, lifestyle changes, or treatments, should always be made **in collaboration with a healthcare professional** who knows your personal medical history.

⚠ I also aim to expose the false promises of miracle cures, quick-fix supplements, and misleading health fads. There is no magic pill, but there is **real, science-backed hope**.

✅ **Change is possible.** And it starts with awareness, knowledge, and action: on your terms, in partnership with your care team.

✏️ A Note on Writing and AI assistance

This book was written with the help of artificial intelligence (AI) as a writing assistant. As someone for whom English is a second language, I used AI to help improve clarity, conciseness, and accessibility of the language. The ideas, structure, and message are fully mine; I stand behind every concept and recommendation presented here.

I believe the future of many fields, including medicine, lies in **human + AI collaboration**. Rather than replacing human insight, tools like AI can enhance communication, accelerate learning, and support better outcomes for both patients and practitioners. There is no reason to hide this process: it's simply a way to produce something clearer, more helpful, and more impactful than would have been possible just a few years ago.

A Bit About Me

To provide some background on the source of this information: I am a primary care physician practicing in Southeast Florida for the past 18 years, with a total of roughly 25 years of experience in primary care. One of the aspects of my work that I cherish most is the long-term relationships I have built with my patients. I often look back at electronic medical records and realize that many of my patients first visited me more than 15 years ago. Some have even brought their children, and in some cases, their grandchildren, to establish care with me. In many ways, this book serves as a general guide for my practice, but also as an opportunity for me to review and deepen my own understanding of these topics.

While I now "walk the talk," I can't claim to have always done so. I know it sounds cliché, so I'll keep my personal story brief. At one point in my life, my activity level was about as sedentary as a couch in storage (yes, a sofa in a living room gets more action). I realized this lifestyle was negatively impacting both the quality and quantity of life. I wasn't feeling well, and I also didn't feel like I had a strong platform to promote healthy habits to my patients. So, about two decades ago, over the course of two years, I lost roughly 70 pounds. I began exercising regularly, became more mindful of my diet, and learned what worked for me: knowledge that I now share daily with my patients.

I don't endorse any specific named diets: there are dozens, if not hundreds, of them, each claiming to be superior. Personally, I am too lazy to restrict my food choices to a single brand, vendor, or set of ingredients. Instead, I advocate for a balanced diet with accessible foods, things we can all find in our local grocery stores without breaking the bank or ordering specialty items online. After my own weight loss, I committed to regular exercise, with a huge influence from my brother-in-law, who encouraged me and patiently waited until my running pace finally started to catch up with his (thank you, Rob!).

Having firsthand experience with weight loss and lifestyle change, I know that writing about it is far easier than doing it. Achieving meaningful results is incredibly difficult, but it is entirely possible. There will be setbacks and moments when progress stalls, but the key is understanding why they happen, accepting them, and getting back on track. Over time, you'll even start to anticipate when setbacks are likely to occur: often, they're diet-related, and you'll gain insight into how to avoid them or recover quickly.

However, since I promised to keep things brief, and this introduction is already getting lengthy, let's get started.

You can connect with the author at:

✉ Email: gabe@gavrimed.com
📷 Instagram: @gabegavrilescu
in LinkedIn: linkedin.com/in/gavrilescumd

CHAPTER 1

Longevity: Science, Trends, and the Future of Lifespan Extension

Defining Longevity

Longevity refers to the length of an individual's life, typically measured as life expectancy at birth or various stages of life. It is a broad concept encompassing genetic, environmental, and lifestyle factors that contribute to an individual's lifespan. While some define longevity simply as an extended life, it is more meaningfully considered as a prolonged period of health and functional well-being, often referred to as "healthspan."

The key focus is not only on extending the number of years lived but also on ensuring those additional years are of high quality, free from debilitating diseases such as cardiovascular disease, cancer, and neurodegenerative disorders.

Biological Fundamentals of Longevity

Longevity is governed by a complex interplay of genetic, cellular, and environmental factors. Biologically, longevity is influenced by several key mechanisms:

1. **Genetic Factors** – Certain genetic variations have been linked to longer lifespans, such as those related to the FOXO3 gene, which plays a role in stress resistance and metabolism regulation (Kenyon, 2010). Studies of centenarians have shown that they often carry protective gene variants that contribute to longevity.

2. **Cellular Senescence and Aging** – Over time, cells accumulate damage due to oxidative stress, DNA mutations, and telomere shortening. Telomeres, the protective caps on the ends of chromosomes, shorten with each cell division, ultimately leading to cellular aging and dysfunction (Blackburn et al., 2015).
3. **Caloric Restriction and Metabolism** – Caloric restriction has been one of the most studied interventions in longevity research. It has been shown to extend lifespan in multiple species by reducing metabolic stress, enhancing autophagy (the body's cellular repair process), and downregulating insulin-like growth factor (IGF-1) signaling (Fontana et al., 2010). Decreasing the activity of IGF-1 has a positive impact on lifespan in animal models (Zhang and Milman, 2022). Lower levels of growth hormone and IGF-1 are associated with increased lifespan in various animal models (Bartke, 2008).
4. **Inflammation and Immune Function** – Chronic inflammation, often referred to as "inflammaging," accelerates aging and contributes to diseases that reduce lifespan. A robust but well-regulated immune system is critical for longevity (Franceschi et al., 2000).

Evolution of Longevity: Trends Over Time

The human lifespan has evolved significantly over millennia. In early human history, life expectancy was around 30–40 years, primarily due to high infant mortality and infectious diseases. However, individuals who survived early childhood could often live into their 60s or beyond.

Key Historical Milestones in Longevity Trends

- **Prehistoric to Ancient Civilizations:** Life expectancy was approximately 30 years due to high rates of infectious disease, malnutrition, and violence.
- **Middle Ages (5th-15th Century):** Life expectancy remained low (~30–40 years) due to plagues, poor sanitation, and limited medical knowledge.
- **18th-19th Century:** The Industrial Revolution brought improvements in sanitation, vaccination, and medical care, leading to a gradual rise in life expectancy (~40–50 years).
- **20th Century:** This century saw the most rapid increase in longevity, particularly in the second half. Advancements in antibiotics, vaccines, public health measures, and medical technology increased life expectancy from approximately 50 years in 1900 to over 75 years by the end of the century (Olshansky & Ault, 1986).

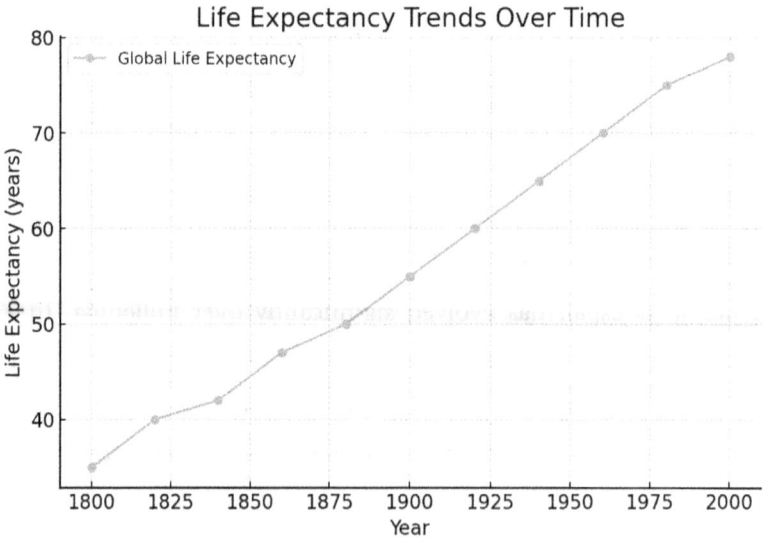

Figure: Global Life Expectancy Trends (1800–2000)

This graph illustrates the steady rise in global life expectancy over the past two centuries, increasing from approximately 35 years in 1800 to nearly 80 years by 2000. This remarkable progress reflects advances in sanitation, medical care, nutrition, and public health.

Longevity in the U.S. vs. the Rest of the World

The U.S. has one of the highest healthcare expenditures per capita, but does not rank among the top countries for longevity. According to recent data, the average life expectancy in the U.S. is approximately 77 years, whereas countries such as Japan, Switzerland, and Singapore have life expectancies exceeding 82 years (World Bank, 2023).

Key Factors Behind Differences in Longevity

- **Diet and Nutrition:** Countries with higher longevity, such as Japan and the Mediterranean nations, have diets rich in whole foods, omega-3 fatty acids, and low processed food consumption.
- **Healthcare Access:** affordable (to individual and country) access to healthcare systems contributes to better preventive care and outcomes (Crowley, 2020).
- **Lifestyle and Physical Activity:** High levels of daily physical activity and social engagement contribute to longer lifespans in countries like Italy and Sweden.
- **Chronic Disease Prevalence:** The U.S. has high rates of obesity, diabetes, and cardiovascular disease, which contribute to lower longevity compared to other high-income nations.

The Role of Social Determinants of Health in Longevity

The following is humbling information for us, physicians, and less well-known and recognized data. Basically, medical care is far from being the main driver of health outcomes. The graph below details the mere 20% of medical care that impacts overall health outcomes, with the rest (80%) being driven by the social determinants of health.

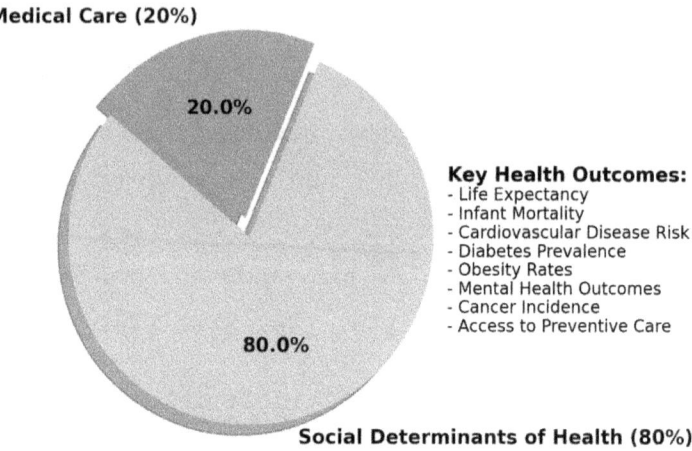

Social determinants of health (SDOH = the conditions in which people are born, grow, live, work, and age) play a far greater role in longevity than medical care alone. Research suggests that social, economic, and environmental factors contribute to approximately 80% of health outcomes, while direct medical care accounts for only about 20% (Magnan, 2017). Key SDOH influencing longevity include income, education, employment, housing stability, food security, and access to healthcare.

For example, individuals with higher education and stable employment tend to experience better health literacy, lower stress, and greater access to preventive care, all of which contribute to a longer lifespan. Conversely, income inequality, food deserts, and inadequate housing contribute to higher rates of chronic disease and shorter lifespans, particularly among marginalized populations. In the U.S., racial and socioeconomic disparities in longevity are stark: life expectancy can vary by up to 15–20 years between affluent and low-income neighborhoods (Chetty et al., 2016).

This gap underscores the fact that longevity is not merely a product of medical advancements, but also of systemic social and economic policies.

Future Trends in Longevity

As medical advancements continue, longevity is expected to rise further. However, disparities in life expectancy between different socioeconomic groups and regions may persist.

Predicted Future Trends:

- **Increased Use of AI and Personalized Medicine:** Artificial intelligence and genomics will allow for highly personalized health interventions.
- **The Role of Cardiovascular Prevention:** Cardiovascular disease remains the leading cause of death worldwide, but advancements in prevention strategies, such as lipid-lowering therapies (e.g., statins), hypertension control, and lifestyle modifications, including enhanced weight management, have significantly improved longevity. Large-scale studies have shown that statins reduce cardiovascular mortality by approximately 25% over five years in high-risk populations (Cholesterol Treatment Trialists' Collaboration, 2019). Their use has contributed to increased life expectancy, particularly in individuals over 50, by reducing heart attacks, strokes, and related complications.
- **Shifts in Dietary and Lifestyle Norms:** Growing awareness of longevity-promoting diets and exercise may help slow aging-related diseases.
- **Economic and Healthcare Challenges:** While longevity may increase, the burden of aging populations on healthcare systems will require policy adjustments.

The Century with the Most Rapid Increase in Longevity

The 20th century saw the most rapid increase in longevity, particularly from 1950 onwards. The combination of improved sanitation, antibiotics, vaccinations, and chronic disease management contributed to a dramatic rise in life expectancy, particularly in developed nations (Cutler & Miller, 2005).

Conclusion

Longevity isn't just a matter of chance: it is shaped by a complex mix of genetics, environment, and lifestyle. While we've come a long way in understanding what helps us live longer and healthier lives, the future of longevity depends on continued research and innovation in healthcare.

On a personal level, the first step to change is to understand the root causes, including genetics. We're all dealt a different hand, but that doesn't mean we're powerless. With the right tools and knowledge, we can shift the odds in our favor and take control of our own risk.

CHAPTER 2

Mortality

Death is inevitable, but how, when, and why we die often reflects far more than biology alone. It tells a story of medical progress, social inequality, access to care, and the lifestyle choices we make every day. Understanding mortality patterns, what kills us, and why, is not just a matter of statistics. It's a gateway to understanding how much control we actually have over our health outcomes and how powerful our decisions can be.

What the Numbers Say

As of the most recent global data, the top causes of death worldwide are dominated by chronic, non-communicable diseases. Ischemic heart disease leads the list, followed closely by COVID-19 and stroke. These three causes alone account for over a third of all global deaths. Chronic obstructive pulmonary disease (COPD) also ranks high. In total, more than 40% of deaths globally are due to just these top four causes.

In the United States, the overall pattern of mortality mirrors global trends, though with some local differences. As of 2023, heart disease remains the leading cause of death, claiming over 680,000 lives. Cancer is a close second, followed by unintentional injuries (accidents), stroke, and chronic obstructive pulmonary disease (COPD). In 2022, COVID-19 was the fourth leading cause of death, but by 2023, it had dropped to tenth. This shift reflects the impact of widespread immunity, improved access to targeted treatments, enhanced preventive strategies, and the circulation of a less virulent viral strain.

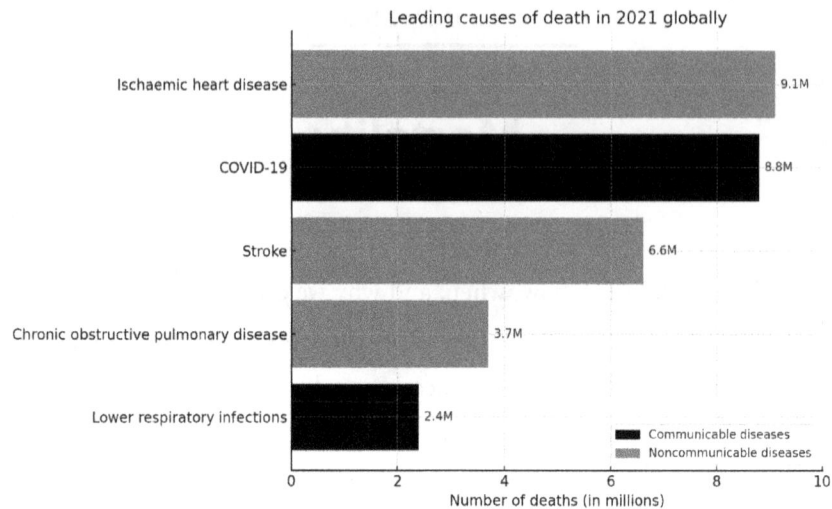

Source: World Health Organization, 2024 - https://www.who.int/news-room/fact-sheets/detail/the-top-10-causes-of-death

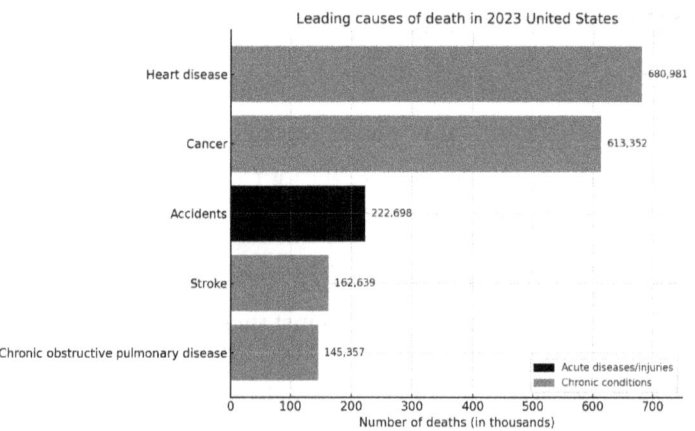

Source: Centers for Disease Control and Prevention, 2023 Provisional Mortality Statistics. CDC Wonder accessed on March 23, 2025 - https://wonder.cdc.gov/controller/datarequest/D176

What's important to remember is that these top causes of death are not random or inevitable. They are deeply connected to modifiable factors, things many of us can influence, like blood pressure, cholesterol, tobacco use, physical activity, vaccination, and diet. And that means there is a real opportunity to shift the odds in our favor.

A Century of Change

Looking back, mortality trends have changed drastically. In 1900, the leading causes of death in the U.S. were infectious diseases like pneumonia, tuberculosis, and diarrheal illnesses. Life expectancy was only about 47 years. However, as public health infrastructure improved, with access to clean water, better sanitation, vaccines, and antibiotics, infectious diseases were gradually brought under control.

From 1900 to 2010, the age-adjusted death rate in the U.S. fell by a stunning 70%, from 2,518 to 747 deaths per 100,000 people. That drop wasn't just due to medical breakthroughs. It reflected deeper societal improvements: education, access to healthcare, nutrition, and public policy.

Today, the mortality burden has shifted to chronic diseases. And unlike infections, these don't typically strike overnight. They build over time, often silently, making prevention both a challenge and an opportunity.

What Drives Modern Mortality?

Cardiovascular Disease

The number one cause of death globally and in the U.S. is cardiovascular disease. Many of its risk factors, like high blood pressure, high cholesterol, diabetes, and smoking, are not only measurable but also modifiable. Yet nearly half of American adults have hypertension, and a striking portion of them are unaware. Even among those treated, **only about 1 in 5 has their blood pressure under control**.

Approximately half (47.3%) of U.S. adults were living with hypertension from 2015 to 2018, and 79.4% of those had uncontrolled hypertension. Of those with uncontrolled hypertension, 70.6% were under age 65 (Vaughan et al, 2022). While almost half of the U.S. population has high blood pressure, 40% of adults with it are unaware, and only 20% of those being treated have it adequately controlled.

Fortunately, progress is being made. Recognition of high blood pressure as a critical risk factor, along with the widespread use of statins (cholesterol-lowering medications), has led to significant reductions in cardiovascular mortality. Studies show that statins not only reduce heart-related deaths but also improve all-cause survival (Orkaby et al, 2020).

There is also strong global evidence supporting the association between higher statin use and lower cardiovascular disease mortality. Countries with greater access to and use of statin medications consistently show reduced death rates from cardiovascular causes, as illustrated in the chart below.

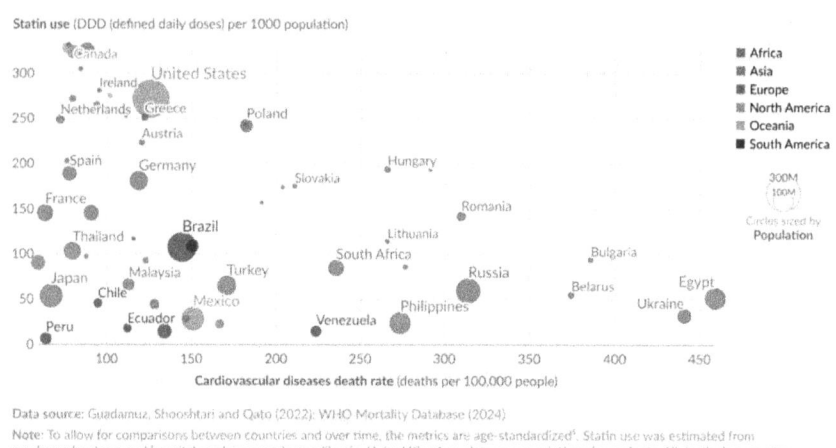

Figure: Relationship between statin use and cardiovascular disease mortality across countries.
Countries with higher rates of statin use per capita tend to have lower cardiovascular death rates, highlighting the role of preventive medication in reducing mortality. Circle sizes represent population size. Source: Guadamuz, Shooshtari, and Qato (2022); WHO Mortality Database (2024).

Cancer

Cancer remains the second leading cause of death, but there's good news here, too. Between 1991 and 2022, cancer mortality in the U.S. dropped by 34%, avoiding an estimated 4.5 million deaths (American Cancer Society, 2025). This progress stems from better screening (breast, colon, cervical, and prostate cancers), more effective treatments, and public health campaigns that dramatically reduced smoking rates.

Decreased rates of tobacco smoking, driven not only by education and health awareness but also by tax policy, advertising restrictions, and local regulations, have played a major role in this favorable trend (Kratzer et al, 2021).

COVID-19

The pandemic reshaped mortality trends in a way we haven't seen in over a century. From 2019 to 2021, life expectancy in the U.S. declined largely due to COVID-19, which accounted for 74% of the drop in 2020 and 50% in 2021. COVID-19 was the third leading cause of death globally by 2021 and remains one of the top five in the U.S. today.

But even here, disparities were highlighted. Communities with less access to care or greater underlying health risks experienced far higher mortality.

A Global Perspective

In low- and middle-income countries, the story is different. While chronic diseases are rising, infectious diseases and maternal and child health issues remain leading causes of death. The reason? Poverty. In many parts of the world, people die not from the lack of a cure, but from the lack of clean water, nutritious food, adequate housing, or basic medical care.

Crowded living conditions, contaminated water, and malnutrition all contribute to higher mortality rates in these regions. These are solvable problems, but solutions require political will, global investment, and grassroots empowerment.

Severe poverty remains the root cause of high mortality in developing countries. It results in malnutrition, inadequate sanitation, overcrowded living, and unsafe water, all of which are entirely preventable conditions.

The Power of Prevention

While the statistics can feel overwhelming, they also point to a hopeful truth: many of the top causes of death are preventable or at least delayable. This book is about taking ownership of the risk factors we *can* control, especially those related to cardiovascular and chronic diseases.

Medical advancements, such as vaccines and antibiotics, have dramatically reduced deaths from infectious diseases. For example, flu vaccination has been shown to have a protective effect against all-cause mortality in older adults (Yedlapati et al., 2021). Improvements in cardiovascular care, such as blood pressure control and the use of statins, have saved countless lives (Virani et al., 2020).

Lifestyle matters. So do screening and early detection. And so does access to care. But even before you walk into a clinic, your daily choices— what you eat, how often you move, whether you smoke or drink— are already shaping your long-term health.

Mortality data isn't just about death. It's about life. It's a mirror, showing us where we've been, where we're vulnerable, and most importantly, where we can go if we choose to act differently.

CHAPTER 3

Drivers of Risk

Before we dive into the details, it's worth saying this clearly: sugar, cholesterol, blood pressure, and weight are not the only things that matter, but they are powerful drivers of risk, and we have simple, effective tools to measure and manage them. Every adult should know their numbers and understand what they mean. That's where primary care providers (PCPs) come in, helping to guide, interpret, and adjust the course when needed. Once you know your values, understand the role they play, and learn how to influence them, you've got a clear and empowering path toward better health, no matter where you're starting from.

Sugar (Glucose)

When we talk about "sugar" as a risk factor, we're not just talking about candy or soda; we're talking about blood sugar, or more precisely, how your body handles glucose over time. It is one of the key drivers for developing diabetes, a condition that can quietly increase your risk for heart disease, stroke, kidney problems, vision loss, and more. Diabetes is defined by high blood sugar.

There are a few common threads among people who develop diabetes. You might be at increased risk if:

- You carry extra weight, especially around your belly
- You don't get much physical activity
- You smoke
- You had diabetes during pregnancy (known as gestational diabetes)
- You have a close relative with diabetes

But here's the thing: not all risk factors are visible, and many people don't feel any symptoms until blood sugar levels are already elevated. That's why I believe in early screening, and not just for those who check all the usual boxes of the risk factors mentioned above.

While different guidelines offer different ages and risk profiles for when to start screening, I prefer a simpler, more inclusive approach: I check everyone's blood sugar levels when they first establish care with me. Why wait until symptoms appear when we can catch early warning signs now?

There are two main tests we use to understand your sugar control:

- Fasting glucose (FPG) – This is your blood sugar level first thing in the morning, after not eating overnight. It's a helpful snapshot.
- A1c (glycated hemoglobin) – This is more of a "movie" than a snapshot. It reflects your average blood sugar over the past 2–3 months, including after meals, during sleep, and throughout daily routines.

Because these two tests measure different things, it's possible to have a normal fasting glucose but a borderline A1c, or vice versa. Both scenarios are important. They don't necessarily mean you have diabetes, but they do suggest your body may be heading in that direction. The sooner we know that, the better our chances of turning things around.

Here's how to interpret your results:

- Normal:
    - A1c < 5.7%
    - Fasting glucose < 100 mg/dL
- Prediabetes:
    - A1c 5.7–6.4%
    - Fasting glucose 100–125 mg/dL

- Diabetes:
  - A1c ≥ 6.5%
  - Fasting glucose ≥ 126 mg/dL in 2 separate instances

If your results are in the normal range, that's great news. I still recommend repeating the test every 1–2 years, just to keep an eye on trends. This is a bit more frequent than what some national guidelines recommend (every 3 years), but in my experience, catching small shifts early allows us to act before bigger problems develop.

The takeaway here is simple: your sugar levels don't define you, but they can inform you. And with that knowledge, you can make powerful choices for your future health.

Cholesterol

Cholesterol is a fat-like substance in your blood that plays essential roles in your body. It helps build cells, produce hormones, and support digestion. Your body is fully capable of making all the cholesterol it needs, with about 80% of it produced by your liver as needed. The remaining cholesterol comes from the foods you eat. Under normal conditions, your body has mechanisms to clear out any extra cholesterol, keeping levels in balance.

But when that balance is off, either because of dietary excesses or because your body isn't able to properly clear cholesterol, levels in the blood can rise, increasing your risk for heart disease and stroke. We check cholesterol levels with a simple blood test called a *lipid panel*, which gives us a snapshot of how your body is handling fats.

Cholesterol gets a lot of attention, and for good reason. It's one of the most important players when it comes to heart disease and stroke risk. But let's clear something up: cholesterol itself isn't the enemy. In fact, your body needs cholesterol to build cells and make hormones. The problem starts when certain types of cholesterol go out of balance or build up in the wrong places, like the walls of your arteries.

There are different kinds of cholesterol, but here are the big three you should know:

- LDL (Low-Density Lipoprotein) – This is often called "bad" cholesterol because it tends to deposit in your arteries, contributing to plaque buildup and narrowing over time. High levels of LDL are strongly linked to heart attacks and strokes.
- HDL (High-Density Lipoprotein) – This is the "good" cholesterol. It helps clear excess cholesterol from your bloodstream and may offer some protection against cardiovascular disease.
- Triglycerides – These are a type of fat in your blood. High levels can also raise your risk for heart disease, especially when combined with high LDL.

You won't feel high cholesterol. There are no symptoms. That's why it's important to check it regularly, usually with a simple blood test called a *lipid panel*. I like to get a baseline on all my patients, regardless of age or health status, especially because some people with "normal" weight and healthy habits still have genetically elevated cholesterol levels.

Fasting or not fasting for the blood draw

There's often confusion about whether a lipid panel needs to be done while fasting. While it used to be standard practice to fast before this test, fasting is usually not necessary, except perhaps the very first time it's being checked. In fact, very few lab tests truly require fasting anymore, despite the idea having been deeply ingrained over the decades.

Most parts of the lipid panel can be accurately interpreted without fasting. The main exception is in individuals with very high triglyceride levels, where fasting may be necessary to obtain an accurate LDL calculation. But for the vast majority of patients, non-fasting labs work just fine (Nordestgaard et al, 2016).

I often see patients delay testing because they can't schedule an early morning appointment, or they try to fast all day just to squeeze in a late-afternoon blood draw, neither of which is necessary in most cases. Unless there's a specific reason to check a fasting glucose, which is a separate test and not part of the lipid panel, **there's no need to fast before getting your cholesterol checked.**

That said, the reverse is also true: **you shouldn't get your labs drawn right after a meal that's very different from your usual routine.** For example, avoid checking your lipid panel the day after a big steakhouse dinner, or right after returning from a vacation or cruise where your eating habits may have been completely out of the norm. In those situations, it's best to wait a few days or longer, depending on the context, so the results reflect your typical lifestyle, not a temporary indulgence.

Here's what a typical lipid panel will measure:

- **Total cholesterol** – Ideally less than 200 mg/dL
- **LDL ("bad") cholesterol** – Ideally less than 100 mg/dL, **but what's considered "normal" varies based on individual specifics.** For some people, especially those without many risk factors, a goal of under 160 or 130 mg/dL may be fine. For others, such as those with diabetes, heart disease, or high overall risk, targets might be 100, 70, or even as low as 55 mg/dL. These decisions are best made in partnership with your doctor, based on your full health picture.
- **HDL ("good") cholesterol** – Ideally above 40 mg/dL for men and above 50 mg/dL for women, though HDL levels are largely driven

by genetics. While it used to be thought that raising HDL would reduce cardiovascular risk, newer research shows that the *number and function of HDL* matter less than previously believed, so hitting your LDL target remains the top priority.

- **Triglycerides** – Ideally less than 150 mg/dL. Elevated triglycerides can be linked to several cardiovascular risk factors, including diabetes, obesity, and diet, particularly excessive intake of refined carbs or high-fat foods (think: a bucket of fried chicken), as well as heavy alcohol use. They can also be elevated due to genetic (familial) causes, which your doctor can help identify and manage appropriately.

There are also two other lab values that are recommended more often and are worth discussing with your doctor:

- **Lipoprotein(a), or Lp(a)** – This is a genetically determined form of cholesterol that correlates with a person's risk of early atherosclerosis (hardening of the arteries). Levels don't change with age, diet, or exercise, so this is something you only need to check once. There's no specific treatment for high Lp(a) at this time, but knowing your level can help better estimate your overall risk.
- **Apolipoprotein B, or Apo B** – This is a protein that helps transport cholesterol in the blood. High levels of Apo B are associated with a higher risk of cardiovascular disease and can provide additional insight into your lipid profile, especially if your LDL or triglycerides are borderline.

The ideal values can vary depending on your personal risk factors. If you've had a heart attack, have diabetes, or have a strong family history of cardiovascular disease, your goals may be even tighter. This is where working with your primary care provider or a cardiologist can really help fine-tune the plan to fit *you*.

The good news? There's a lot you can do to improve your cholesterol. Diet, exercise, weight management, and sometimes medication (like statins) all play a role. But the first step is **knowing your numbers** and understanding what they mean for your health.

Just like with blood sugar, having elevated cholesterol doesn't mean something's broken; it just means it's time to act. When you understand how to improve your numbers and reduce your risk, **you take control of your future health, one step at a time.**

Blood Pressure

Blood pressure is the force your blood exerts against the walls of your arteries as your heart pumps it around your body. It naturally rises and falls throughout the day, affected by stress, activity, sleep, and emotions. But when it stays elevated over time, it silently damages your arteries and vital organs. That's why it's often called the "silent killer."

You won't feel high blood pressure. There are no warning signs. You can feel completely fine, yet still be at risk. That's why regular, accurate monitoring is so important.

A blood pressure reading consists of two numbers:

- The top number (systolic) measures pressure when your heart beats;
- The bottom number (diastolic) measures pressure when your heart rests between beats.

A healthy reading is usually less than 120/80 mmHg. Here's a basic guide:

- Normal: Less than 120/80 mmHg
- Elevated: Systolic 120–129 mmHg and diastolic less than 80 mmHg
- Stage 1 Hypertension: Systolic 130–139 mmHg or diastolic 80–89 mmHg
- Stage 2 Hypertension: Systolic ≥140 mmHg or diastolic ≥90 mmHg

That said, **blood pressure targets can shift depending on age and overall health.** In older adults, especially those in their 80s and 90s, systolic readings in the 140s or even 150s, and diastolic readings in the high 80s to low 90s, may be acceptable. That's because stiffening of the artery walls that occurs naturally with age can lead to higher readings that aren't necessarily harmful. In these cases, aggressively lowering blood pressure could actually do more harm than good.

These values are intended as general guidelines, not "one-size-fits-all" rules. The right target for you should be determined in partnership with your doctor, taking into account your age, overall health, medications, and personal risk factors. **Nothing replaces a face-to-face conversation with a trusted physician.**

But here's something most people don't realize: blood pressure readings can vary significantly, even from moment to moment. That's why *how* and *where* the reading is taken matter just as much as *what* the numbers are.

I will include a detailed description in the '*How The Damage Can Be Undone or Prevented*' chapter on how to check blood pressure accurately at home.

Weight

Obesity is a major risk factor for many of the chronic conditions we're trying to prevent: heart disease, stroke, diabetes, and even some types of cancer. It's a complex issue, deeply connected to both individual biology and the world we live in.

Weight is commonly assessed using **Body Mass Index (BMI)**, which is calculated by dividing a person's weight in kilograms by the square of their height in meters (kg/m^2). While not a perfect measurement, BMI helps categorize weight ranges for adults into general categories recognized by the World Health Organization:

- **Underweight:** BMI < 18.5
- **Normal weight:** BMI 18.5–24.9
- **Overweight:** BMI 25–29.9
- **Obesity:** BMI ≥ 30
- **Severe obesity:** BMI ≥ 40

Obesity is now considered one of the leading causes of premature death worldwide. And it's not just a personal challenge; it's a societal one. Over the past century, changes in our food systems, environments, and lifestyles have tilted the scales. We're surrounded by calorie-dense, processed foods. Physical activity has taken a backseat to screen time, long commutes, and sedentary jobs. And all of this has consequences.

Back in the early 1960s, just 13% of American adults were classified as obese, according to data from the CDC. Today, that number is closer to 43%.

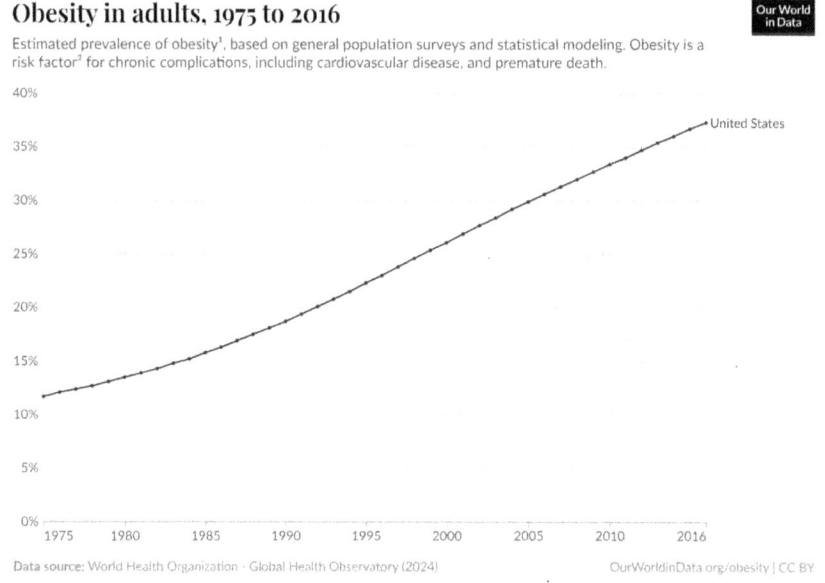

In the United States, obesity rates have tripled since the 1960s to the present, and, even more concerning, rates of severe (or "morbid") obesity have increased tenfold over that same period (USAFacts).

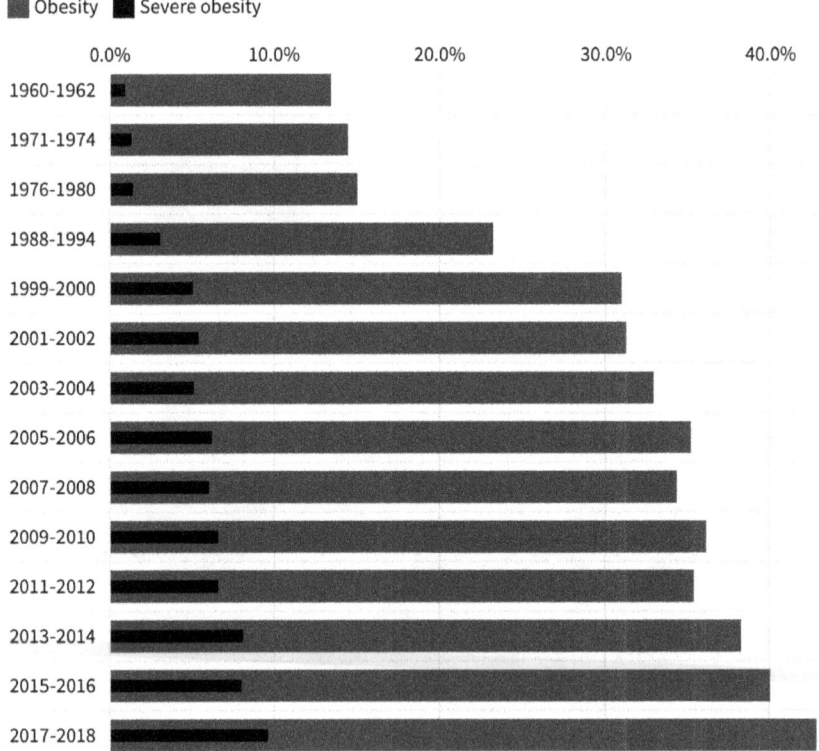

From a medical perspective, weight gain occurs when energy intake (calories eaten) exceeds energy expenditure (calories burned) (Guyton and

Hall, 2021). That part is straightforward. But what drives that imbalance is far more complex. There are multiple overlapping contributors, including genetics, hormones, sleep, medications, stress, and the environment in which people live.

Yes, genetics plays a significant role. Some people store fat more easily than others. Some lose weight quickly; others struggle. It's not just about willpower, it's about biology. This is why two people can eat similarly and move similarly but end up with very different outcomes. This is not a blame game. **Every patient deserves to be understood within the context of their own life, health history, and environment. There's much more to weight than food choices alone.**

Social determinants of health also heavily influence obesity trends. According to the CDC, disparities in obesity rates across the country may be explained by systemic factors such as:

- Lower high school graduation rates
- Higher unemployment
- Food insecurity and lack of access to healthy, affordable food
- Limited spaces for safe physical activity
- Targeted marketing of unhealthy products
- Poor access to healthcare or community support systems

Age also plays a role. As we get older, our metabolism slows down, and our bodies require fewer calories, but often we continue to eat the same amount or more. At the same time, we tend to lose muscle mass and become less active, both of which contribute to weight gain. For women, hormonal changes after menopause can shift fat distribution, often increasing abdominal fat due to declining estrogen levels.

So while the formula of "eat less, move more" is technically true, **it's an oversimplification** of a deeply layered issue. The goal here isn't to shame anyone into change; it's to understand the science, recognize the many influences at play, and provide support and strategies that are realistic, respectful, and rooted in health, not just numbers on a scale.

CHAPTER 4

How the Damage is Done

Heart Attack / Stroke

When we hear about someone having a heart attack or a stroke, it often sounds sudden and unexpected. But the truth is, these events are usually the *final chapter* of a long, silent process unfolding inside the body, sometimes over years or even decades. At the heart of it is a condition called atherosclerosis.

Atherosclerosis is the gradual buildup of plaque, a mix of fats, cholesterol, inflammatory cells, and other materials, inside the arteries. Over time, this buildup causes the arteries to narrow and stiffen, limiting blood flow to vital organs. But the real danger often comes when a plaque ruptures. That rupture can trigger a clot, which may completely block the artery. When this happens in the heart, it causes a heart attack (medically known as a myocardial infarction). When it happens in the brain, it leads to a stroke.

But how does this process begin?

It all starts with an injury to the endothelium, the thin inner lining of your blood vessels. This lining is normally smooth and protective, but when it's damaged by high blood pressure, high blood sugar, or low-density lipoprotein (LDL) particles, it becomes more vulnerable. LDL particles, especially when oxidized, play a key role in initiating inflammation in the artery wall. The injured area becomes "stickier," attracting more LDL and white blood cells, which leads to further inflammation and growth of the plaque.

As the plaque builds, the artery narrows, silently restricting blood flow. Eventually, a piece of plaque breaks off, a clot forms, and an organ is suddenly starved of oxygen. That's the brief description of the process behind a heart attack or a stroke.

And it's not just the heart and brain that are at risk. Atherosclerosis can affect the kidneys, limbs, and other organs. But because heart attacks and strokes are the most common and deadly outcomes, they're often the focus of prevention efforts, and rightly so.

The Role of Cholesterol: What Research Shows

A strong body of scientific literature supports the critical role of cholesterol, particularly the LDL subfraction of cholesterol, in the development of cardiovascular disease. Here's a look at three major studies that help paint the picture:

- A meta-analysis (a type of study that combines data from many individual studies to draw stronger conclusions) involving over 1 million participants found that higher levels of total cholesterol and LDL-C (low-density lipoprotein cholesterol) were significantly associated with increased mortality from cardiovascular disease (Jung et al, 2022).
- Another large-scale study with over 2.5 million participants showed that elevated cholesterol levels in young adults were linked to a higher risk of developing cardiovascular disease later in life. Importantly, individuals who lowered their cholesterol levels saw a reduced risk of future heart and vascular problems (Jeong et al, 2018).
- A landmark genetic and clinical evidence review published in *The European Heart Journal* concluded that LDL is not just associated with, but causally linked to atherosclerosis. This consensus statement underscored that "the lower the LDL, the better" when it comes to reducing the risk of heart attacks and strokes (Ference et al, 2017).

The Role of Tobacco: A Dangerous Double Threat

Smoking is one of the most potent and well-established contributors to heart attack and stroke risk. It harms the cardiovascular system in two major ways. First, it introduces toxic chemicals and carcinogens that directly damage the endothelium (the delicate lining of the blood vessels), accelerating the development of atherosclerosis. Second, smoking increases systemic inflammation, disrupts healthy cholesterol levels, and elevates blood pressure.

Even light or occasional smoking can have measurable effects on cardiovascular risk, and secondhand smoke isn't harmless either. The good news? The benefits of quitting start almost immediately: within weeks, blood pressure improves, circulation begins to recover, and the risk of heart attack begins to decline. Long-term, quitting smoking can cut cardiovascular risk in half in 3-6 years after tobacco cessation (CDC, 2020).

The Role of Alcohol: More Isn't Better

Alcohol's relationship with cardiovascular health is complex, but heavy or chronic use clearly raises the risk for both heart attacks and strokes.

Alcohol can raise blood pressure, promote arrhythmias (irregular heart rhythms), and increase levels of triglycerides in the blood. It may also impair liver function and contribute to weight gain, diabetes, and inflammation, all of which feed into the atherosclerosis process. For strokes, particularly hemorrhagic (bleeding) strokes, alcohol is an especially strong risk factor.

Some studies have suggested that low to moderate alcohol intake (particularly red wine) might have cardiovascular benefits, but this remains controversial, and the protective effect, if any, is far outweighed by the harm of regular or high-volume drinking. For prevention, less is more, and for many, no alcohol at all is the safest path forward.

So, What Does This Mean for You?

It means that managing cholesterol, alongside other risk factors like tobacco use and alcohol consumption, isn't just about improving lab numbers. It's about preventing the actual damage that leads to life-altering events like heart attacks and strokes.

The earlier we act, the more we can do to keep our arteries clean, our organs nourished, and our futures protected.

Diabetes

Diabetes is defined by elevated levels of glucose in the blood. The body regulates blood sugar through the action of insulin, a hormone produced by the pancreas. Throughout this book, when I refer to diabetes, I'm focusing on what's classically known as type 2 diabetes, also called adult-onset diabetes.

Type 1 diabetes, by contrast, is an autoimmune disorder in which the body's immune system mistakenly attacks and destroys the insulin-producing cells in the pancreas. It's typically diagnosed earlier in life, often during childhood or adolescence, and is characterized by a near-total absence of insulin.

Type 2 diabetes, on the other hand, involves insulin resistance, where the body still produces insulin, but the cells no longer respond to it properly. This form develops gradually and is far more common.

As glucose levels begin to rise, the condition is often asymptomatic. It doesn't come with alarms or sudden pain. Instead, it tiptoes quietly, sometimes for years before an official diagnosis.

Unless caught early, it can cause real and lasting damage. But here's the empowering truth: type 2 diabetes is largely preventable, and even after diagnosis, it can often be well-controlled. With the right lifestyle changes and medical guidance, many people can bring their blood sugar back into a safe, near-normal range, dramatically reducing the risk of complications and restoring long-term health.

From Insulin Resistance to Diabetes: The Silent Progression

The story often begins with insulin resistance. Insulin is a hormone your body produces to help move glucose from your bloodstream into your cells, where it can be used for energy. But over time, especially when we carry excess visceral fat (fat stored deep in the abdomen), lead sedentary lives, and consume diets high in refined carbs and added sugars, our cells start to become resistant to insulin's signal.

In response, the pancreas tries to compensate by pumping out more insulin. This works for a while, but eventually, the system gets overwhelmed. Blood sugar begins to rise, first into a range known as prediabetes, and then into type 2 diabetes. All the while, many people feel completely fine. That's why diabetes is often called a *silent disease*: you may not notice anything until complications begin to surface.

Why Blood Sugar Becomes Toxic

Our bodies are designed to maintain blood sugar levels within a tight, healthy range. When sugar levels remain elevated over time, it begins to damage tissues, especially small blood vessels and nerves.

Think of your blood vessels (especially the inner lining, called the endothelium) as a smooth, protective surface guiding the flow of blood. Now imagine if, day after day, tiny grains of sandpaper were dragged along that surface. That's what chronically high blood sugar can do. It doesn't rip or tear things open in one dramatic moment, but it *gradually scours the surface*, wearing it down, making it rough, inflamed, and more prone to plaque buildup and clots.

This microscopic irritation disrupts the endothelium's function: it can't dilate properly, loses its anti-inflammatory properties, and begins to signal for help, attracting inflammatory cells. Over time, this contributes to atherosclerosis, the same process behind heart attacks and strokes. And because small blood vessels are especially fragile, they're often the first to suffer.

- In the eyes, this leads to retinopathy, one of the leading causes of blindness.
- In the kidneys, it can lead to nephropathy, eventually causing kidney failure and the need for dialysis if glucose levels are not controlled in the long term.
- In the nerves, high glucose levels impair signaling, leading to neuropathy, which is often characterized by burning, tingling, or numbness, particularly in the feet.
- In the extremities, narrowed arteries and damaged nerves can lead to poor wound healing, infections, and amputations if glucose remains uncontrolled in the long term.
- And in the heart and brain, elevated blood sugar accelerates plaque buildup, increasing the risk of heart attacks and strokes.

These aren't random complications; they're connected consequences of sugar's wear and tear on the vascular system.

Cancer

Cancer can feel like one of the most unpredictable and frightening diagnoses. And while it's true that not all cancers are preventable, we now know that many are influenced by factors we can control, things like lifestyle habits, infections, environmental exposures, and our body's internal chemistry.

Data from the Global Burden of Disease Study estimated that in 2019, over 50% of cancer deaths in men and more than one-third in women were linked to behavioral, environmental, occupational, or metabolic risk factors (Tran et al, 2022). That's a powerful reminder that cancer isn't always just bad luck; sometimes, it's the result of a long-standing imbalance in the body, often decades in the making.

Let's take a closer look at the most common and modifiable contributors to cancer risk.

Inflammation: The Hidden Spark

One of the lesser-known drivers of cancer is chronic inflammation. While inflammation is part of the body's natural healing response, persistent inflammation, especially in the presence of metabolic stress, toxins, or infection, can damage cellular DNA, increasing the likelihood of mutations that lead to cancer. Over time, this inflamed environment creates fertile ground for abnormal cells to grow and spread.

One of the mechanisms through which this happens is mitochondrial dysfunction. Mitochondria, the powerhouses of the cell, are not only responsible for generating energy but also play key roles in regulating cell death, DNA repair, and cellular signaling. When mitochondria become damaged or dysfunctional (often due to oxidative stress, aging, or metabolic imbalance), they can produce excessive reactive oxygen species, which directly harm cellular DNA. This increases the risk of mutations, genomic instability, and uncontrolled cell growth, all hallmarks of cancer. Additionally, impaired mitochondrial function can disrupt normal cellular apoptosis (programmed cell death), allowing potentially cancerous cells to survive and proliferate.

Infections That Trigger Cancer

Several infections have a direct link to cancer, particularly in regions with limited access to vaccines or early treatment:

- HPV (Human Papillomavirus): Associated with cervical, anogenital, and head and neck cancers.
- HBV (Hepatitis B virus): Strongly linked to liver cancer.
- HIV (Human Immunodeficiency Virus): Raises the risk for several cancers, including certain lymphomas.
- Helicobacter pylori: A common bacterium associated with gastric cancer.

Vaccination, screening, and treatment of these infections represent important, and often overlooked, opportunities for cancer prevention.

Tobacco: Still the Biggest Offender

Tobacco remains one of the most potent carcinogens known to medicine. Half of all smokers will die from a tobacco-related disease. Its connection to lung cancer is well known, but it also increases risk for cancers of the mouth, throat, bladder, pancreas, and more.

Tobacco causes cancer through a double assault: direct injury from carcinogens and the promotion of chronic inflammation. It's not just about what's in the smoke, it's about what it does to the cells and tissues it touches, day after day.

Physical Inactivity and Cancer Risk

You may not think of exercise as a cancer prevention tool, but it's one of the most consistent protective factors we have. Regular physical activity has been shown to reduce the risk of several types of cancer, colon and breast cancer being among the most well-studied (Inoue et al, 2008). Movement helps regulate hormones, reduce inflammation, and improve immune surveillance, all of which contribute to lower cancer risk.

Alcohol and Cancer: The Dose Matters

Alcohol consumption, especially in excess, has been linked to increased risk for oral, esophageal, breast, and colorectal cancers. Studies show a dose-response relationship: the more alcohol consumed, the higher the cancer risk (Rumgay et al, 2021; Praud et al, 2016; Xi et al, 2017). That means even modest reductions in alcohol intake may offer protective benefits.

Excess Weight and Metabolic Risk

In the United States, it's estimated that 40% of all cancers are associated with excess weight (Gallagher et al, 2015). And this isn't just about body size, it's about what's happening *inside* the body.

Conditions such as obesity and type 2 diabetes are characterized by insulin resistance and hyperinsulinemia (excessive circulating insulin), both of which are linked to higher levels of insulin-like growth factor (IGF-1). This hormone promotes cell growth, and when left unchecked, may fuel tumor development and progression.

Other metabolic changes common in obesity and diabetes, like chronic inflammation, altered gut microbiota, and dysregulated lipids, also appear to increase cancer risk. What's more, these abnormalities often begin *years* before diabetes is officially diagnosed, meaning the window for prevention is wider than many people realize.

Estrogen also plays an important role. In individuals with excess body fat, particularly postmenopausal women, adipose tissue becomes a primary site of estrogen production. Elevated estrogen levels have been linked to a higher risk of hormone-sensitive cancers, especially breast and endometrial cancer. This is one of the reasons why maintaining a healthy body weight is so important for cancer prevention.

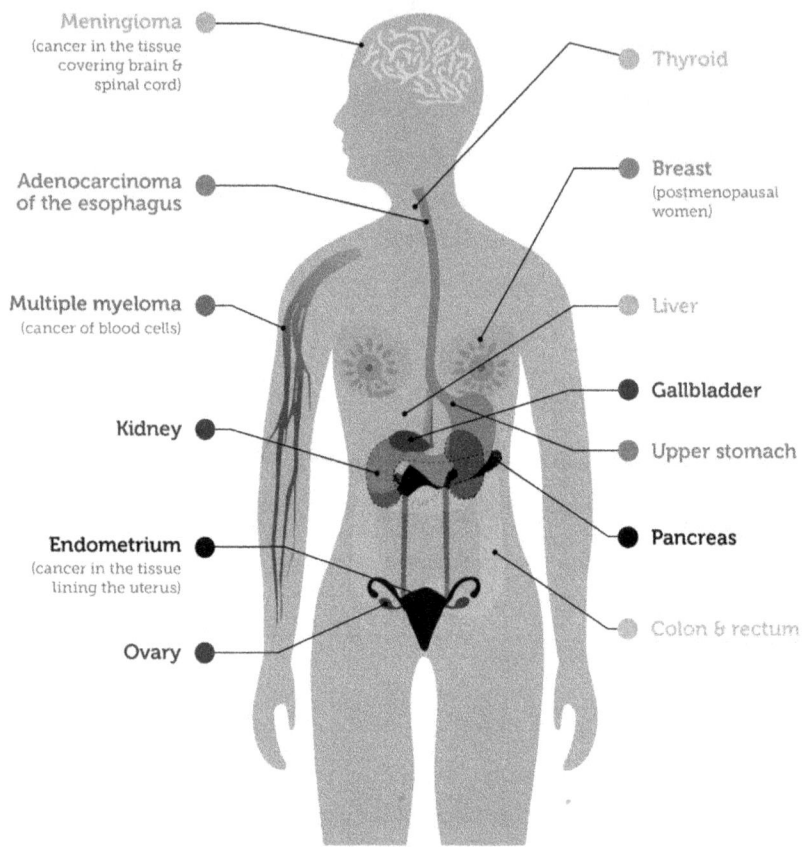

Cancers associated with being overweight or obese.
Source: National Cancer Institute (NCI)

Cancer can be complex and multifactorial, but it's not entirely out of our hands. The same lifestyle choices that protect your heart and brain—reducing inflammation, managing weight, staying active, avoiding tobacco, and limiting alcohol consumption— **also build a strong defense against many of the most common cancers.**

Dementia

Brain Health Is Strongly Linked to Overall Body Health

When it comes to memory and cognition, many of us are particularly attuned to our family history. If a parent or sibling has been diagnosed with dementia, we often seek extra screenings, second opinions, or reassurance, and that's completely understandable.

About 25% of adults age 55 and older have a first-degree relative (a parent, sibling, or child) with dementia (Loy et al, 2014). And while the lifetime risk of developing dementia in the general population is around 10%, that number doubles to 20% for those with a family history.

But let's flip that number around.

In my "glass is more than half full" view, that also means 80% of people with a family history *won't* go on to develop dementia. That's a powerful statistic, and it leads us to an important truth: while we can't change our genetics, we can absolutely change our risk.

Looking Beyond Genetics: What We *Can* Control

When it comes to dementia, **atherosclerosis** - yes, the same process we discussed in the heart attack and stroke section - plays a starring role. While there are many forms of dementia, this book focuses on what you can do to protect your brain, rather than breaking down every subtype in detail.

The two most common causes of dementia are:

- **Alzheimer's disease**, which is marked by the buildup of **amyloid plaques** in the brain
- **Vascular dementia**, caused by reduced blood flow to brain tissue due to narrowed or blocked arteries

In reality, many people have **both** processes occurring at once, a situation known as **mixed dementia**. It's common, and it reflects just how deeply **vascular health and brain health** are intertwined.

With vascular dementia, the same plaque that clogs arteries in the heart can build up in the brain's blood vessels, limiting oxygen and nutrient delivery. When that blockage causes a stroke in a large enough region, memory can decline sharply and suddenly. But more often, small vessel disease is at play: Plaque builds up in the brain's smaller arteries, impairing blood flow bit by bit. The result is a gradual decline in memory, thinking, and processing speed, less dramatic than a stroke, but just as meaningful over time.

Chronic inflammation is another shared thread. Whether triggered by high blood sugar, smoking, excess weight, or hypertension, inflammation fuels both vascular damage *and* neurodegeneration. It acts like a low-grade fire in the body, one that can slowly damage blood vessels, impair healing, and disrupt the normal function of brain cells over time.

And the same culprits keep showing up: high blood pressure, elevated cholesterol, diabetes, smoking, and inflammation. These risk factors silently damage the vascular system for years before any symptoms appear.

The Case for Early Action: Risk Factors in Midlife Matter

Here's the really hopeful part: many of the risk factors that contribute to dementia are already present and detectable in midlife, sometimes even earlier.

One large study followed more than 15,000 adults between the ages of 44 and 66 for 25 years. It found that several common conditions were associated with a higher risk of dementia later in life (Gottesman et al, 2017):

- Diabetes (Hazard Ratio: 1.8)

- Smoking (HR: 1.14)
- Hypertension (HR: 1.4)
- Prehypertension (HR: 1.3)

Let's pause for a second to explain the term **hazard ratio (HR)**. In simple terms, it compares the risk of an event (like dementia) between two groups. An HR of 1.8 means the risk is **80% higher** in one group compared to another. It doesn't mean everyone with diabetes will develop dementia, but it does mean they're at **significantly increased risk**.

And the risk adds up. In another study, people with three or more risk factors, such as diabetes, smoking, hypertension, and heart disease, had a hazard ratio of 3.4 for Alzheimer's disease (Luchsinger et al, 2005). That's more than a threefold increase.

Modifiable Risk Factors That Protect the Brain

- Regular physical activity
- Healthy diet (Mediterranean/DASH-style)
- Blood pressure control
- Cholesterol management
- Stress reduction & quality sleep
- No smoking
- Limit alcohol
- Weight management
- Blood sugar control (prevent or reverse prediabetes/diabetes)

The Special Link Between Diabetes and the Brain

Diabetes alone is associated with a 1.5 to 2 times higher risk of dementia (Livingston et al, 2017), and studies suggest that poorer glucose control, as measured by hemoglobin A1c (HbA1c), further increases that risk (Avadhani et al, 2015).

The mechanisms behind this are still being studied, but here's what we know so far:

Beyond its cardiovascular effects, diabetes also appears to interfere with how the brain clears amyloid, the sticky protein that forms the plaques characteristic of Alzheimer's. The brain produces a small amount of its own insulin, and in diabetes, especially with long-term insulin resistance, this brain insulin may be reduced, impairing amyloid clearance.

Amyloid is a normal protein found throughout the body, but when it accumulates excessively in the brain, it can disrupt communication between neurons, trigger inflammation, and ultimately contribute to the memory loss we associate with Alzheimer's disease.

Why This Matters

Dementia is not a fate sealed by genetics alone. Yes, family history plays a role, but so do decades of lifestyle, metabolic health, and cardiovascular care. And the earlier we act, the more room we have to prevent or delay decline.

So, let's focus on the part we *can* control. Your brain is not separate from your body. Your arteries, your blood sugar, and your pressure all affect your memory. And the same healthy habits that support your heart can also help keep your mind sharp for decades to come.

The vicious circle linking all: the metabolic complex of diseases

Let's take a moment to recap what we've covered so far in this chapter. We've seen how heart attacks and strokes are driven by atherosclerosis, high LDL cholesterol, inflammation, diabetes, and high blood pressure. We explored type 2 diabetes, which often begins with insulin resistance and progresses silently in the context of increased weight. We discussed how cancer risk rises in the setting of inflammation, insulin resistance, and excess weight. And we examined how dementia and cognitive decline often trace back to those same culprits: atherosclerosis, insulin resistance, and chronic inflammation.

Across all of these, we saw how tobacco, alcohol, and lack of physical activity act as accelerators, fueling the underlying processes that lead to damage.

- Tobacco increases inflammation, introduces toxic substances, worsens blood pressure, and contributes carcinogens directly linked to cancer.
- Alcohol raises glucose and blood pressure, promotes weight gain, and creates both direct inflammation and toxic effects on organs.
- Sedentarism (too little movement) amplifies weight gain, worsens insulin resistance, and promotes inflammation, contributing meaningfully to heart disease, dementia, diabetes, and cancer.

Lack of physical activity has been called "the new smoking." A landmark study (King, 2012) proposed that sedentarism may carry a similar level of health risk as smoking because both behaviors significantly raise the odds of coronary artery disease, diabetes, certain cancers, and premature death. When smoking and sedentarism coexist (as they often do), the effects are even more damaging.

A large number of the conditions that define metabolic syndrome are deeply tied to a sedentary lifestyle.

What Is Metabolic Syndrome And Why Don't More People Know About It?

Metabolic syndrome is a cluster of conditions, often symptom-free, that together significantly raise the risk for cardiovascular disease and other chronic illnesses. The concept is well known in the medical community, but far less recognized by the general public. And part of that problem, I believe, lies in how we've defined it.

There's no single, universally accepted definition. At least five different medical associations have proposed slightly different criteria. While there's a fair amount of overlap between them, the lack of one clear, consistent standard has made this condition harder for patients to understand and easier to overlook.

For the purposes of this book, I've chosen the most practical and accessible version: the definition provided by the National Cholesterol Education Program Adult Treatment Panel (NCEP ATP III). According to this guideline, a person is diagnosed with metabolic syndrome if they meet three or more of the following five criteria:

1. Fasting glucose $\geq$ 100 mg/dL, or currently on medication for diabetes
2. Low HDL cholesterol (< 40 mg/dL in men, < 50 mg/dL in women)
3. Triglycerides $\geq$ 150 mg/dL
4. Abdominal obesity (waist circumference > 102 cm in men or > 88 cm in women)
5. Blood pressure $\geq$ 130/85 mmHg, or currently on medication for hypertension

Even this "simplified" version can be hard to digest, with gender-based cutoffs and the inclusion of HDL and triglycerides, markers that, while valuable, are less familiar to most people. Personally, in my day-to-day practice, I often focus on LDL > 130 mg/dL as a more actionable, widely recognized starting point for patient education. I'm fully aware that LDL isn't part of the formal diagnostic criteria, and that HDL and triglyceride values have their known value in risk. Still, it's a simplification that helps make the discussion more tangible for patients.

Metabolic Complex of Diseases: A Broader View

The term "metabolic syndrome" itself is also limiting. It focuses only on cardiovascular and diabetes risk but leaves out two of the most important modern health threats: cancer and dementia.

That's why I propose we begin thinking in terms of the **Metabolic Complex of Diseases**, an evolved concept that acknowledges a shared root system linking these four major chronic conditions:

- Atherosclerosis → Heart attacks, strokes, dementia
- Insulin resistance → Type 2 diabetes, cancer, dementia, heart attacks, strokes
- Chronic inflammation and obesity → Cancer, heart attacks, strokes
- Vascular and metabolic dysfunction → Dementia, heart attacks, strokes

The diagram below illustrates the complex, interconnected web of cause and effect between these conditions. They don't exist in isolation; *they feed each other*, amplify one another, and often share the same modifiable risk factors.

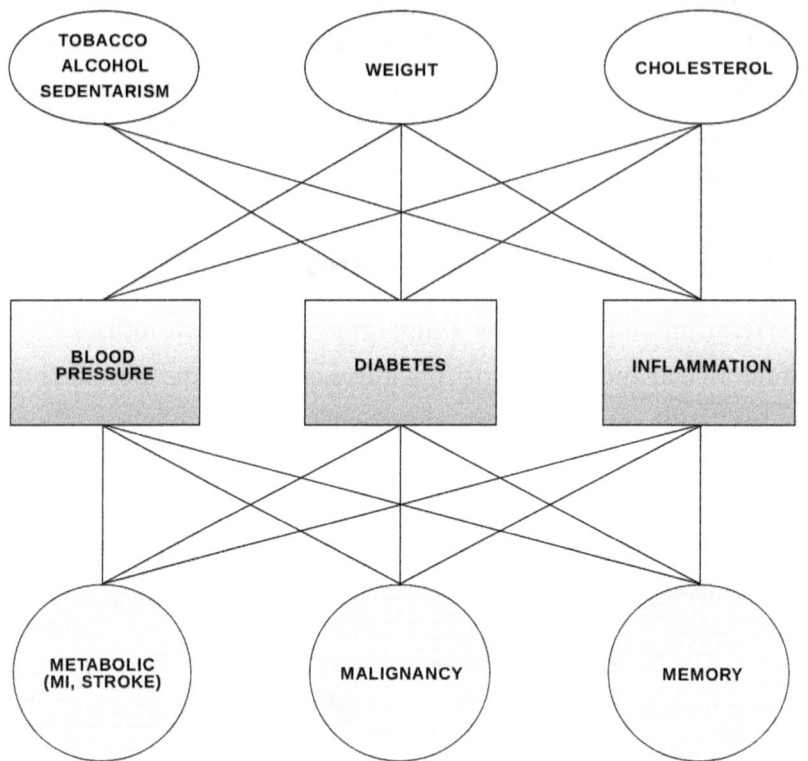

And the stakes are enormous.

Together, these four conditions, atherosclerosis (including heart attacks and strokes), cancer, dementia, and diabetes, along with hypertension, accounted for over 1.7 million deaths in the United States in 2023, according to Centers for Disease Control and Prevention data (CDC, Leading Causes of Death, 2023). That's 55% of all deaths in the country. Put another way, **more than 1 in every 2 deaths is tied to this web of interlinked diseases.**

What's Missing from the Definitions?

Surprisingly, there's still no officially defined syndrome linking metabolic syndrome and dementia, despite an overwhelming body of research showing their strong connection. This lack of recognition may be why many people overlook the opportunity for prevention, opting instead for over-the-counter "brain boosters" with no evidence of benefit, often promoted in celebrity-endorsed commercials.

These products may generate hundreds of millions of dollars in revenue, but they offer little (if any) help. Imagine the impact if even a fraction of that money were redirected toward public education on managing blood pressure, cholesterol, glucose levels, and promoting physical activity. The truth is simple: *there is no magic pill.* But there is a powerful formula: eat well, move often, manage stress, stay engaged, and take care of your numbers.

Likewise, there's no formal syndrome connecting metabolic dysfunction and cancer, despite growing literature showing how insulin resistance, obesity, and inflammation fuel certain cancers, worsen progression, and alter outcomes (Pothiwala et al., 2009).

While I'm not in a position to create formal medical terminology (that's far beyond my expertise and role), I would like to propose the term **M3 Complex of Diseases (Metabolic, Memory, Malignancy)** for the purposes of this book, as a way to more accurately and clearly capture the interconnected nature of these conditions.

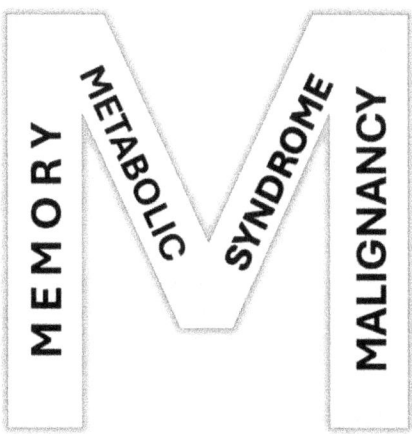

It's Time to Think Differently

The framework of the M3 Complex of Diseases invites us to zoom out, to stop looking at each disease in isolation and instead recognize the common seed from which they grow. It gives us a clearer path forward: by managing the upstream drivers, we can influence a broad spectrum of outcomes.

This is where prevention becomes both practical and powerful. And it begins with awareness.

Let's stop thinking of **health** as a collection of separate problems and start seeing it for what it really is: **an interconnected system**, where even small improvements in lifestyle can ripple across the entire body and across generations.

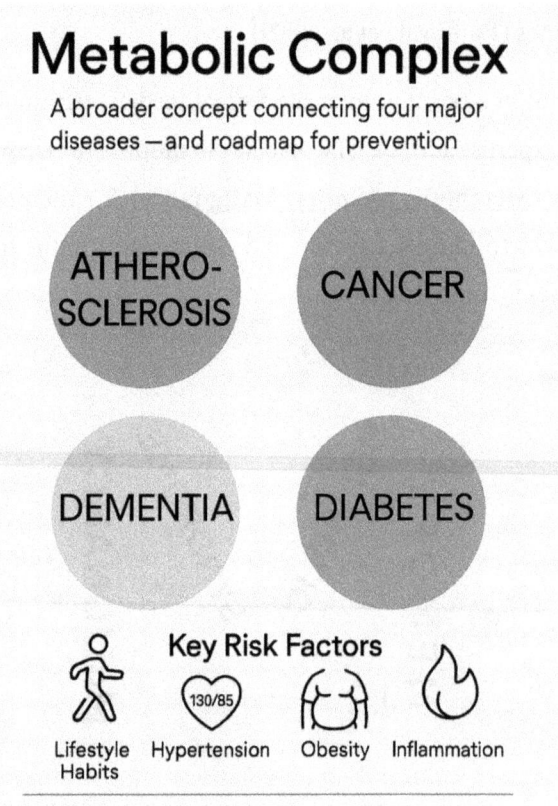

CHAPTER 5

How the Damage Can Be Undone or Prevented: Diet, Exercise, Tobacco and Alcohol Avoidance

Diet

Let's start this chapter, the "how" of reducing M3 risk, with the one modifiable factor that most people wrestle with: diet. In the first part of the book, we explored the "why," the foundational causes behind the diseases grouped under M3 (metabolic, malignancy, memory). Now, we move to the "how": what we can actually do to tilt the balance in our favor.

The Merriam-Webster dictionary offers several definitions of "diet":

- food and drink regularly provided or consumed,
- habitual nourishment,
- the kind and amount of food prescribed for a special reason,
- a regimen of eating and drinking sparingly to reduce weight.

The first two refer to our typical, unrestricted dietary patterns, the kind of diet I'd personally love to follow every day without limits, but that I try to steer away from based on what I've learned and experienced. Realistically, I still slip into that default mode from time to time, and that's okay. These lifestyle shifts are not about perfection. They're aspirational, not absolute. We're human. There will be ups and downs.

The third definition is "prescribed for a special reason," that is what I'd call a healthy, balanced diet. One that supports weight maintenance and metabolic health when weight loss isn't needed. Think: Mediterranean diet. The fourth definition, eating and drinking sparingly, is the classic weight-loss regimen. And yes, this is the harder one to follow, but it's also the one we'll focus on more, especially in the DIY chapter later.

In regions known as "Blue Zones," people routinely live longer, healthier lives, often attributed in large part to dietary patterns:

- **Okinawa, Japan:** Many live beyond 100, attributed to plant-based meals, time-restricted eating, physical activity, and close social bonds.
- **Nicoya Peninsula, Costa Rica:** High life expectancy is associated with a diet rich in whole, unprocessed foods, particularly beans, fruits, vegetables, and whole grains, combined with an active lifestyle and strong family support.
- **Sardinia, Italy:** Longevity in this region has been linked to the Mediterranean diet and regular physical activity.
- **Ikaria, Greece:** Known for its tight-knit community, afternoon naps, low stress, and a diet rich in plants, olive oil, and fish, contributing to remarkably low rates of chronic diseases and cognitive decline.

Are you wondering why they're called "Blue Zones"? No poetic meaning, just that the researchers who first identified these regions (led by Dan Buettner) happened to circle them in blue marker color on the map.

Back to our own grocery carts and meal plans: there are hundreds of diets out there, many with flashy marketing, monthly fees, or specialized ingredients. My approach is more pragmatic: basic cooking skills, minimal grocery store wandering, and certainly no subscription plans. I'm building an approach for someone like me and maybe like you: frugal, busy, and looking for practical, science-backed, sustainable choices.

At the core of any weight-loss plan is a simple yet powerful principle: **create a safe and sustainable calorie deficit**. In other words, **eat fewer calories than you burn**. That's what leads to gradual, healthy weight loss. But as you've likely experienced, real life makes that difficult. Between family meals, holidays, business lunches, and snacks at every turn, it's easy for intake to exceed output. Modern society has further complicated things by normalizing the idea of three full meals plus multiple snacks daily, a pattern reinforced over the past century by aggressive messaging from the food industry. Yet for thousands of years, human beings followed a very different rhythm. The hunter-gatherer model involved eating when food was available, not on a fixed schedule, and certainly not five or six times a day. Despite the lack of constant access to meals, our ancestors not only survived but thrived, physically active and resilient, without chronic disease. It's only in recent history that abundance has quietly become one of our greatest challenges.

How to Calculate One's Caloric Needs?

How many calories should be in one's diet? It depends on the calories that are burned, i.e., the energy expenditure. It also depends on age, weight, and gender.

First, we need to know the basal metabolic rate (BMR). It is a formula I am adding here but there is no need to bother with it as you can add that into any search engine or AI tool to get the particular result for a particular individual.

BMR (men)= 10 × weight (kg) + 6.25 × height (cm) − 5 × age (years) + 5

BMR (women)= 10 × weight (kg) + 6.25 × height (cm) − 5 × age (years) − 161

To understand caloric needs better, think of your body like a car:

- **Your Basal Metabolic Rate (BMR)** is like a car idling at a red light; it's the minimum amount of fuel your engine needs just to stay running. That's your body at rest, keeping your heart beating, lungs breathing, and brain conducting the entire 'orchestra'.
- **Your Total Daily Energy Expenditure (TDEE)** is what happens when you start driving. How much fuel you burn depends on whether you're cruising gently or racing up a hill. TDEE accounts for your BMR *plus* everything else you do: walking, exercising, digesting food, even fidgeting.

TDEE = BMR × Activity Factor (AF), where:

- Sedentary (little or no exercise): AF= 1.2
- Lightly active (light exercise/sports 1-3 days/week): AF= 1.375
- Moderately active (moderate exercise/sports 3-5 days/week): AF=1.55
- Very active (hard exercise/sports 6-7 days/week): AF=1.725
- Extra active (very hard exercise/sports and physical job): AF= 1.9

For example, a 52-year-old man, 98 kg, 200 cm, exercising moderately:

- BMR ≈ 1,975 kcal/day
- TDEE ≈ 3,061 kcal/day

That's his maintenance calorie level. Eating below that level consistently will lead to gradual weight loss. Here's the challenge: **we tend to underestimate what we eat and overestimate what we burn.**

Fortunately, technology helps. Apps that scan barcodes or log meals can teach us about portion sizes, calories, and hidden ingredients. You only need a few weeks of consistent tracking to build a good sense of how different foods affect your body and your weight trends.

People often say, "I eat healthy but can't lose weight." And they might be right, kind of… Home-cooked meals and healthy ingredients still carry calories, and if you eat too much of them, weight loss won't happen. Portion size matters. The goal is to align what goes in with what's burned, doing so without compromising nutritional quality.

What Makes a Diet "Healthy"?

We can simplify dietary composition into three key macronutrients:

- Protein
- Carbohydrates
- Fat

For weight loss, maintaining adequate protein intake is especially important. It supports metabolism, helps preserve muscle mass, and increases satiety.

A healthy diet isn't just about eating less; it's about eating smart. That means balancing your **macronutrients**:

- **Proteins** help preserve muscle mass, support metabolism, and increase satiety.
- **Carbohydrates** fuel your body and brain, but should be chosen wisely (favor complex over refined).
- **Fats** play important roles in hormone regulation, cell structure, and nutrient absorption.

For most people aiming to lose weight, maintaining a **daily protein intake of 1.0 to 1.4 grams per kilogram of body weight** is a solid target. Don't worry, later in the DIY section, I'll show simple ways to estimate this without needing a calculator or a food science degree. No need to memorize how many grams of protein are in every type of fish or poultry. Thankfully, we live in 2025, and smart tools can do the heavy lifting.

Let's now review some of the most well-studied diets, those that promote general health, metabolic control, or intentional weight loss.

> 📌 **A Quick Note on Calories vs. Kilocalories**
>
> Throughout this book, you may notice the terms *calories* and *kilocalories (kcal)* used interchangeably. Technically, **1 kilocalorie (kcal)** equals **1,000 calories (cal)**-the amount of energy needed to raise the temperature of 1 kilogram of water by 1°C. However, in the context of nutrition and food labeling, **"calorie" almost always refers to a kilocalorie**. When you see a food label stating "200 calories," it really means 200 kilocalories. This is a widespread convention, and for readability, I follow the same approach in this book.

The Mediterranean Diet

This is often held up as the gold standard of healthy eating. The Mediterranean diet emphasizes:

- Fruits and vegetables
- Whole grains
- Legumes and nuts
- Olive oil as the primary fat source
- Moderate amounts of fish and poultry
- Minimal red meat and sweets

Macronutrient breakdown:

- **Protein**: 15–25%
- **Carbohydrates**: 45–65%
- **Fat**: 25–35%

Evidence supports its impact across the entire M3 spectrum. A large meta-analysis of 40 trials with over 35,000 participants at elevated cardiovascular risk found that those adhering to the Mediterranean diet had a lower risk of all-cause mortality and heart attacks. Stroke risk was also reduced (Karam et al., 2023). Another study, conducted in Spain, confirmed that individuals who followed a Mediterranean diet had fewer heart attacks, strokes, and cardiovascular deaths compared to those on a low-fat diet (Delgado-Lista et al., 2022).

Even more impressively, it's linked to **reduced rates of Alzheimer's, Parkinson's**, and several cancers, including prostate, breast, and colorectal (Sofi et al., 2008; Schwingshackl et al., 2014; Toledo et al., 2015). The overlap is no coincidence; this dietary pattern targets the upstream causes of M3 diseases.

Paleo Diet

The paleo approach is inspired by what humans are believed to have eaten during the Paleolithic era. It emphasizes:

- Meat and fish
- Fruits and vegetables
- Nuts and seeds

It excludes:

- Grains
- Dairy
- Legumes
- Processed foods and sugars

Macronutrient breakdown:

- **Protein**: 30%
- **Carbohydrates**: 35%
- **Fat**: 35%

Paleo diets often promote weight loss and reduced intake of processed foods, but long-term adherence and data on broader disease prevention are more limited.

Ketogenic Diet

Keto takes a different route: by dramatically lowering carbohydrate intake and increasing fat, the body is pushed into **ketosis**, using fat (instead of glucose) for fuel. Common foods include:

- Fatty fish
- Eggs
- Cheese
- Meats
- Non-starchy vegetables

Macronutrient breakdown:

- **Protein**: 20–25%
- **Carbohydrates**: 5–10%
- **Fat**: 70–75%

In clinical practice, I've noticed many patients on keto experience significant increases in **LDL cholesterol**. I can often guess when someone has started a ketogenic diet just by looking at their lab results.

Currently, we lack strong long-term data to support the benefits of the ketogenic diet for metabolic or cardiovascular health in the general population.

That said, it's important to acknowledge that **keto does have a well-established role in the medical management of certain seizure disorders**, particularly in individuals with epilepsy that hasn't responded to other treatments. While that specific use falls outside the scope of this chapter, it serves as a reminder that every diet has a context, and what works therapeutically for one condition may not always be suited for broader health goals.

Vegan Diet

A vegan diet eliminates all animal products and includes:

- Fruits
- Vegetables
- Whole grains
- Nuts
- Legumes and seeds

Macronutrient breakdown:

- **Protein**: 15–25%
- **Carbohydrates**: 50–60%
- **Fat**: 20–30%

This diet has been associated with lower risks of heart disease, diabetes, high blood pressure, and some cancers. It's also beneficial for **LDL cholesterol** and **triglycerides**. However, it requires careful attention to **vitamin B12**, **iron**, and **protein sources**. I recommend annual lab checks for those on strict vegan diets.

Observational studies suggest that plant-based diets are associated with lower risks of obesity, heart disease, diabetes, hypertension, certain cancers, and decreased all-cause mortality (Orlich et al., 2013; Barnard et al., 2009).

Low-Carb Diet

Low-carb diets, including Atkins, limit carbohydrate intake while increasing protein and fat. While similar to keto, they are typically **less extreme** and more flexible.

Macronutrient breakdown:

- **Protein**: 30–40%
- **Carbohydrates**: 10–30%
- **Fat**: 30–40%

These diets often lead to short-term weight loss, but depending on the sources of protein and fat (especially if rich in saturated fats), they may increase **LDL cholesterol** and cardiovascular risk. Long-term evidence is mixed, and some observational studies suggest **higher mortality rates** when animal proteins and saturated fats dominate the plate (Seidelmann et al., 2018).

Low-Fat Diet

Low-fat diets reduce total fat intake and emphasize:

- Lean proteins
- Whole grains
- Fruits and vegetables
- Low-fat dairy

Macronutrient breakdown:

- **Protein**: 20–25%
- **Carbohydrates**: 55–65%
- **Fat**: 10–25%

This diet reduces **saturated and trans fats**, which can help lower LDL cholesterol levels and reduce the risk of heart disease. It's also commonly used in clinical guidelines for weight management and cardiovascular prevention.

DASH Diet

The **DASH** diet (Dietary Approaches to Stop Hypertension) was developed to help lower blood pressure. It emphasizes:

- Fruits and vegetables
- Whole grains
- Lean proteins
- Low-fat dairy
- Limited sodium, sugar, and red meat

Macronutrient breakdown:

- **Protein**: 18%
- **Carbohydrates**: 55%
- **Fat**: 27%

While it doesn't replace the need for blood pressure medications in most individuals, it works synergistically with them. Studies show DASH may also reduce the risk of colorectal cancer, cardiovascular events, and premature mortality (Schwingshackl et al., 2017), though its impact on **overall mortality** isn't as well-established as the Mediterranean diet.

Intermittent Fasting (IF)

Unlike the diets above, intermittent fasting isn't about what you eat, but when. It focuses on timing, cycling between periods of eating and fasting. Common patterns include:

- **16:8** – Fast for 16 hours, eat in an 8-hour window
- **5:2** – Eat normally 5 days/week; limit calories on 2 days

- **Alternate-Day Fasting** – Rotate eating and low-calorie days (~ 500 kcal/day)
- **24-hour fasts** – Once or twice a week, no food for a full day

IF has gained traction for its ability to reduce **inflammation**, improve **insulin sensitivity**, and assist with **weight loss**.

Before starting any form of intermittent fasting, it's important to first have a conversation with your primary care doctor. While many people can follow this approach safely, especially with the right motivation, certain individuals may be more vulnerable, particularly those prone to low blood sugar or with a limited ability to produce glucose from internal stores. For them, fasting could lead to uncomfortable or even concerning symptoms. That said, most people adapt surprisingly well once they ease into it.

The early stages may feel challenging, but the body learns to adjust. When intermittent fasting is combined with one of the healthy dietary patterns discussed earlier, it can have synergistic effects, reducing inflammation, improving insulin resistance, and supporting sustained weight loss. A study by de Cabo et al. (2019) found that intermittent fasting can improve metabolic health and even slow aging. Mattson et al. (2018) noted benefits for brain health, including animal studies showing a delay in Alzheimer's and Parkinson's disease progression. More recently, Liu et al. (2023) showed intermittent fasting supports weight loss, lowers blood sugar, enhances insulin sensitivity, and activates autophagy. Think of autophagy as a kind of cellular 'spring cleaning' that helps repair damage and slow disease.

Importantly, populations like **Okinawans** naturally follow intermittent fasting-like eating schedules and show some of the lowest rates of obesity, diabetes, and cardiovascular disease in the world.

The table below summarizes the above diets and their impacts on the main triggers of the M3 group of diseases.

Diet	Protein	Carbohydrates	Fat	LDL Effect	Insulin Resistance	Inflammation	Sustainability	Evidence Strength
Mediterranean	15-25%	45-65%	25-35%	Decreases	Improves	Reduces	High	Strong
Paleo	30%	35%	35%	Neutral/Variable	Improves	Reduces	Moderate	Moderate
Ketogenic	20-25%	5-10%	70-75%	Often Increases	Improves	May Increase	Low	Limited (Long-term)
Vegan	15-25%	50-60%	20-30%	Decreases	Improves	Reduces	Moderate to High	Moderate
Low-Carb	30-40%	10-30%	30-40%	Often Increases	Improves (short-term)	Variable	Moderate	Mixed
Low-Fat	20-25%	55-65%	10-25%	Decreases	Improves	Reduces	High	Moderate
DASH	18%	55%	27%	Decreases	Improves	Reduces	High	Strong
Intermittent Fasting	Varies	Varies	Varies	Improves	Improves	Reduces	Moderate	Emerging

Foods That Promote vs. Hinder Healthy Aging

We've explored how different diets can support weight loss and reduce M3-related risks, but it's equally important to look at specific food groups, not just entire diet patterns. The quality of what we eat every day has a profound impact on how we age, on our energy, memory, cardiovascular function, and resilience to disease.

A 2025 study published in *Nature Medicine* (Tessier et al. 2025) highlighted that **plant-based diets**, low in processed foods and sodium, especially when adopted in midlife, significantly promote healthy aging. These diets were linked to preserved cognition, reduced risk of chronic disease, and maintained physical function well into older age. The conclusion was simple: your food choices today shape your health decades from now.

So, what should we lean into and what should we limit?

✓ Foods That Promote Healthy Aging

Food Group	Examples
Fruits	Berries, apples, oranges
Vegetables	Leafy greens, broccoli, carrots
Whole Grains	Brown rice, quinoa, oats, bulgur, whole wheat bread
Unsaturated Fats	Olive oil, avocados, fatty fish
Nuts & Legumes	Almonds, walnuts, lentils, peas, kidney beans
Low-Fat Dairy	Skim milk, yogurt, low-fat cheese

These foods are rich in fiber, antioxidants, healthy fats, and phytonutrients. They support immune function, reduce inflammation, lower blood pressure, and help maintain cholesterol balance. Unsaturated fats, especially **monounsaturated fats (MUFA)** from nuts, seeds, and olive oil, are particularly important in protecting heart and brain health.

A helpful tip at the grocery store: **liquid fats at room temperature** (like olive or canola oil) are usually the healthy ones (MUFA), while **solid fats** (like butter or lard) are typically saturated fats (SFA) and should be limited.

✘ Foods That Hinder Healthy Aging

Food Component	Examples
Trans Fats	Packaged snacks, pastries, some margarines
High-Sodium Foods	Canned soups, deli meats, fast food
Sugary Beverages	Sodas, sweetened fruit drinks, energy drinks
Red & Processed Meats	Bacon, sausages, hot dogs, salami, bologna
Ultra-Processed Foods	Instant meals, frozen entrées, shelf-stable snacks

The principle is simple: **the more processed a food is, the more likely it is to harm your health**. If your grandmother wouldn't recognize it as food, think twice. The more a food is altered from its original state through the addition of additives, preservatives, artificial flavors, or chemical stabilizers, the less likely it is to support long-term health. **Trans fats**, often hidden in processed snacks and baked goods, are especially harmful, as they increase inflammation and are strongly linked to cardiovascular disease. **Processed meats** like bologna, sausages, and hot dogs are associated with increased risks of diabetes, stroke, and certain cancers, particularly those affecting the gastrointestinal tract (Abete et al., 2014; Kaluza et al., 2012; Feskens et al., 2013).

Whenever possible, it's best to choose foods that are **closer to their natural form**: whole, minimally processed, and made with ingredients you can easily recognize and pronounce. This simple shift toward real, recognizable food can make a significant difference in preventing the chronic conditions that so often follow in the footsteps of a modern, ultra-processed diet.

Sugary beverages are especially sneaky. A single 8-ounce glass of orange juice contains roughly 110 calories, about twice the amount of a whole orange, but without the fiber. If you're drinking sweetened beverages throughout the day, those "empty calories" add up fast. For a 180-pound person, it takes about **30 minutes of walking at a moderate pace just to burn 150 calories.**

And what about artificial sweeteners? While they technically don't contain calories, they can trick the brain by separating sweet taste from actual caloric content. This can interfere with appetite regulation and increase cravings. Some studies show that people who regularly consume artificially sweetened beverages may end up compensating by eating more overall, ironically leading to weight gain. In fact, the World Health Organization now recommends against the routine use of non-sugar sweeteners for weight control, citing a lack of long-term benefit.

A Final Word on Berries

Among fruits, **berries** deserve a special shout-out. They're nutrient powerhouses:

- **Blueberries** have been linked to a lower risk of diabetes, improved cognitive function, and heart health.
- **Raspberries** are high in fiber and low in sugar, making them ideal for weight-conscious eaters.
- **Blackberries** offer anti-inflammatory benefits and are rich in vitamin C and K.
- **Strawberries** support immune function and are packed with antioxidants.
- **Acai berries** have antioxidant properties, being rich in vitamins A and C
- **Cranberries** also have strong antioxidant properties and are commonly used to reduce urinary tract infection symptoms.

Despite their natural sweetness, most berries are relatively low in sugar. **Half a cup** contains about **40–50 calories**, a great return on investment for such a small, nutrient-dense portion. Just remember: moderation still matters, especially if you are monitoring blood sugar or total caloric intake.

Diet is the cornerstone of disease prevention and healthy aging, nourishing the body with what it needs while minimizing what accelerates damage.

It plays an outsized role in determining weight, metabolic balance, and long-term health. In fact, when it comes to weight loss specifically, **diet is responsible for an estimated 80–90% of the effort**, with exercise contributing the remaining 10–20%. But food is only part of the equation. Just as we are what we eat, we are also how we move.

The benefits of physical activity extend far beyond burning calories: it improves insulin sensitivity, strengthens cardiovascular health, enhances brain function, and may even lower the risk of cancer.

In the next section, we'll explore how movement works hand-in-hand with nutrition to support and sustain health, and why **exercise is one of the most powerful tools we have** in undoing or even preventing the damage caused by the M3 spectrum of diseases.

Exercise

Let's start with a common misconception: the role of exercise in weight loss. It's certainly important, but when we zoom in on the numbers, **diet does the heavy lifting**, accounting for about 80 to 90% of weight loss outcomes. Exercise makes up the remaining 10 to 20%.

There's a saying that captures it well: **"Weight loss happens in the kitchen, and maintenance happens in the gym."**

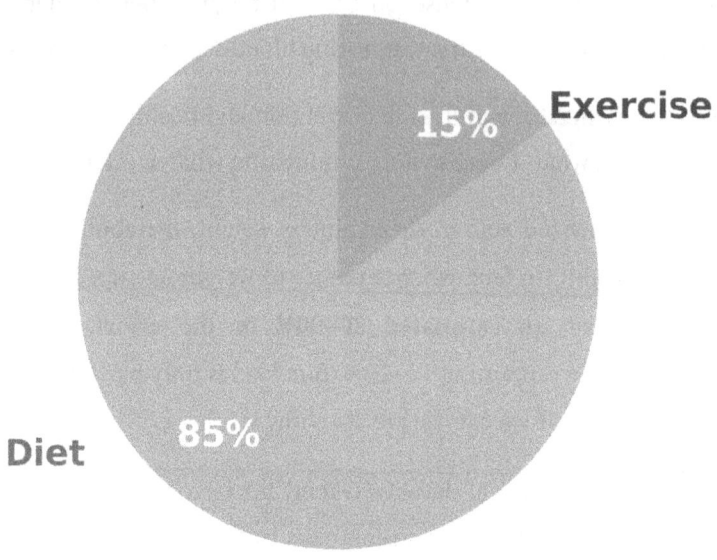

Contribution to Weight Loss: Diet vs. Exercise
"Weight loss happens in the kitchen, and maintenance happens in the gym"

That doesn't make movement optional, though. In fact, the true value of physical activity lies in what happens beneath the surface. Regular movement helps regulate insulin, reduces chronic inflammation, enhances brain resilience, lowers blood pressure, and improves lipid profiles. It's a critical lever in maintaining the weight we've lost, preserving muscle mass, and keeping the body metabolically flexible. And perhaps most importantly, it supports physical and mental well-being in ways that go far beyond the scale.

If diet is the cornerstone of disease prevention, exercise is its most powerful ally. It's one of the few interventions that benefits all three components of M3: **metabolic, malignancy, and memory**. Like diet, physical activity has a far-reaching impact. And in many cases, a single habit, like a daily walk, can tackle more than one target at once. It's not just common knowledge that exercise helps; there's overwhelming scientific evidence to support it.

Regular physical activity is associated with a significant reduction in all-cause mortality, regardless of age, gender, body type, or starting fitness level. In one large-scale prospective study involving over 250,000 adults aged 50 to 71, adherence to national physical activity guidelines led to striking results:

- Moderate activity (30 minutes most days of the week) reduced mortality risk by 27%.
- Vigorous activity (20 minutes, three times a week) was linked to a 32% reduction.
- Those who met both guidelines saw a 50% lower risk of death.

Importantly, even individuals who exercised less than the recommended amount experienced a 19% reduction in mortality risk compared to completely inactive individuals (Leitzmann et al., 2007).

This is a message that deserves emphasis: **any movement is better than none**, and the benefits start earlier than many people think. There's no age threshold, no weight requirement, and no fitness prerequisite to begin. Too often, people give up on exercise because they don't meet a particular goal, especially weight loss.

That brings us to a critical misconception: the belief that exercise must lead to weight loss to be worthwhile. I often see individuals abandon physical activity because the scale doesn't budge after a few weeks of workouts. But as discussed earlier, **exercise contributes only 10–20% to weight loss efforts**. Its value lies far beyond the number on the scale.

In fact, **fitness may be more important than weight**. A comprehensive meta-analysis (Barry et al., 2014) covering over 800 studies found that unfit individuals had double the risk of mortality compared to those who were fit, regardless of BMI. In other words, **a normal-weight person who is unfit** has a **higher risk of death** than someone who is overweight but physically fit. Similarly, **overweight and obese individuals who were fit from a cardiorespiratory point of view** had **mortality risks similar to their normal-weight, fit peers.**

This is not just academic. A recent 2024 study by Weeldreyer et al. reinforces the message: cardiorespiratory fitness remains one of the strongest predictors of survival, and it attenuates the risks associated with being overweight or obese.

The takeaway? **Don't let the scale determine your motivation to move.** As these studies suggest, we should shift our mindset from focusing solely on weight loss to promoting **physical activity as a primary intervention** to reduce mortality risk. This shift in focus could change the way we approach not only public health, but our personal habits, too.

Unfitness, not body weight, is the more pressing risk. Fortunately, the remedy is simple and available to almost everyone: **move more, sit less, and find a routine that you can stick with**. The body and brain respond to that consistency with resilience, improved function, and a longer life.

	Normal BMI	Overweight / Obese
Fit	Low Risk	Low Risk
Unfit	High Risk	High Risk

What Type of Exercise Is Recommended?

Let's take a look at the official guidelines from the CDC for adults aged **18 to 64**:

- Aerobic activity:
    - 150–300 minutes per week of moderate-intensity (e.g., brisk walking), or
    - 75–150 minutes per week of vigorous-intensity (e.g., running, HIIT)

- Muscle-strengthening:
    - Activities involving all major muscle groups at least 2 days per week

For adults 65 and older, the recommendations remain the same, but they may need to be adapted to individual health conditions and physical abilities. In addition, there's an emphasis on balance training, especially to reduce the risk of falls, with Tai Chi routine being one well-studied and accessible option.

But here's the key message: **any exercise is better than none.**

Even if you can't meet the full guidelines every week, occasional movement still delivers meaningful benefits.

A 2023 study by Inoue et al. looked at step count data from U.S. adults and found that walking 8,000 steps or more, even just 1–2 days per week, was associated with a significant reduction in both all-cause and cardiovascular mortality over a 10-year period. The benefit was not exclusive to daily walkers. The data showed that step counts between 6,000 and 10,000 also reduced risk, even if performed intermittently. This is especially encouraging for people with demanding schedules who may not be able to meet daily goals.

Another large study by Saint-Maurice et al. (2020) reinforces this message:

- Walking 8,000 steps/day = 51% lower mortality risk than walking 4,000 steps/day
- Walking 12,000 steps/day = 65% lower mortality risk than 4,000 steps/day
- Interestingly, step intensity (speed or pace) was not associated with lower mortality; step count mattered more.

With the wide availability of wearable devices, including pedometers in most smartphones and smartwatches, it's easier than ever to track your steps and set small, achievable targets. Even a simple reminder to take a walk at lunch or park a bit farther away can add up. And now we have the data to prove that it really does count.

What Happens at the Cellular Level (Mitochondria)

Mitochondria are the **microscopic power plants** housed inside nearly every cell in the body. Their primary function is to generate the energy that cells require to function. But their role doesn't stop there: mitochondria are also key players in aging, inflammation, and oxidative stress, all of which contribute to cellular damage and chronic disease, as discussed earlier in the book.

Insulin resistance impairs mitochondrial function, weakening the body's ability to use energy efficiently and increasing cellular stress. However, the process is reversible. Improving insulin sensitivity can help repair cells and stimulate the creation of new mitochondria, a process known as mitochondrial biogenesis.

One of the most powerful effects of exercise, beyond anything visible on the scale, is its ability to enhance insulin sensitivity. When we move our muscles, especially during moderate to vigorous activity, they begin to absorb glucose from the bloodstream more effectively, and they require less insulin to do so. Over time, this repeated demand for **energy helps reverse insulin resistance**, a root cause of **metabolic syndrome and type 2 diabetes**.

At the cellular level, **exercise improves both the quantity and quality of mitochondria**. The better these mitochondria function, the more efficiently the body can burn both glucose and fat for fuel. In individuals with insulin resistance, mitochondrial dysfunction is common, but regular physical activity helps **rebuild this energy system**, restoring metabolic flexibility and reducing chronic inflammation.

In short, movement doesn't just burn calories, it reprograms your cells to function better.

And here we find yet another shared root among the diseases in the M3 group: cellular impairment and repair. Whether we're talking about metabolic dysfunction, inflammation, cognitive decline, or cancer, mitochondria are involved. In fact, dementia is increasingly being linked to insulin resistance, which is tightly connected to poor mitochondrial function. When mitochondrial health suffers, so does cellular performance in the brain and across the entire body.

A clear and consistent relationship exists between fitness levels and the risk of dementia. A large UK study by del Pozo Cruz et al. (2022) involving over 78,000 participants found that **daily step count was strongly linked to dementia risk in a nonlinear fashion.**

This means that the risk doesn't decrease at a perfectly steady rate with every additional step; instead, the greatest gains occur early, with substantial risk reduction seen even at lower step counts, and the benefits taper off as step numbers continue to rise.

Taking around **9,800 steps per day** appeared to offer the **greatest protection**, but even as few as **3,800 steps daily** was associated with a **25% reduction in dementia risk.**

Importantly, this study also highlighted the role of stepping intensity and peak 30-minute cadence, not just total steps, suggesting that purposeful movement may be especially beneficial for brain health. This differs slightly from studies on mortality, where the total number of steps mattered more than the pace. Still, the core message remains: **more movement means better brain health.**

The connection may lie, once again, at the cellular level, specifically within the mitochondria. Mitochondrial dysfunction plays a critical role in fostering neurodegenerative processes, including those seen in dementia (Monzio Compagnoni et al., 2020). When mitochondria become impaired, there is more oxidative stress, which in turn damages DNA and disrupts normal cellular function. This not only contributes to cognitive decline but also increases the risk of malignancy. Recent research has shown that altered mitochondrial function can affect the tumor microenvironment, impair immune surveillance, and allow cancer cells to evade detection (Wang et al., 2023).

In summary, maintaining mitochondrial health is essential, not just for energy production but for preserving brain function, preventing inflammation, and protecting against cancer. The best tools we have to support our mitochondria are regular physical activity, a balanced diet, and a lifestyle that favors movement over sedentary behavior. These choices aren't just about feeling good in the short term; they're about changing your risk trajectory for the long term.

A large study involving over 1.4 million individuals (Moore et al., 2016) found that leisure-time physical activity is associated with a lower risk of many types of cancer. The authors define leisure-time activity as:

"Activities done at an individual's discretion to improve or maintain fitness or health."

The study demonstrated a linear relationship between physical activity and cancer risk, meaning that the more you move, the lower your risk. Specifically, higher levels of activity (≥6 METs) were associated with significantly lower risks for a wide range of cancers, including:

- Esophageal, liver, lung, kidney, gastric, endometrial,
- Myeloid leukemia, multiple myeloma,
- Colon, head and neck, rectal, bladder, and breast cancer.

The table below provides examples of physical activities and their corresponding **MET (Metabolic Equivalent of Task) intensities**, as outlined by Haskell et al. in the 2007 article *"Physical Activity and Public Health."*

Light Intensity (<3.0 METs)	Moderate Intensity (3.0–6.0 METs)	Vigorous Intensity (>6.0 METs)
Sitting at a desk (1.5 METs)	Brisk walking (3.3–4.0 METs)	Running at 6 mph (9.8 METs)
Playing cards (1.5 METs)	Vacuuming or mopping (3.0–3.5 METs)	Swimming laps (freestyle, 5.8 METs)
Walking slowly (2.0 METs)	Bicycling at 10–12 mph (6.0 METs)	Jumping rope (12.3 METs)
Billiards (2.5 METs)	Tennis doubles (5.0 METs)	Soccer (competitive, 10.0 METs)
Playing musical instruments (2.0–2.5 METs)	Golf (walking, pulling clubs, 4.3 METs)	Basketball game (8.0 METs)

Interestingly, the study by Moore also noted a higher incidence of prostate cancer and malignant melanoma among more active individuals. The researchers suggest that this may be due, in part, to greater health surveillance, as physically active individuals are more likely to attend routine screenings, which could lead to earlier detection of otherwise indolent conditions like prostate cancer.

As for the higher incidence of malignant melanoma, the likely explanation is increased sun exposure during outdoor activities. This serves as an important reminder, especially for runners, hikers, and outdoor enthusiasts, to take **sun protection seriously**.

- Apply sunscreen regularly
- Wear UV-protective clothing
- Schedule routine skin checks with a dermatologist

Malignant melanoma is the most dangerous form of skin cancer. It arises from pigment-producing cells and has the potential to spread rapidly if not detected and treated early.

The benefits of exercise in reducing cancer risk are supported by a growing body of research. One such study, published by McTiernan et al. (2018), not only confirms this protective effect but also highlights that in individuals already diagnosed with breast, colorectal, or prostate cancer, increased physical activity is associated with a 40–50% reduction in both all-cause and cancer-specific mortality.

Let's pause on that for a moment. Imagine a medication that could cut your risk of dying from cancer by half and achieve that with no major side effects. That's the power of exercise. To put it another way: if 100 individuals have cancer, and 20 of them are expected to die over a certain period, adding exercise to the mix could reduce that number to just 10. That's a profound shift in outcome, driven by something entirely within reach.

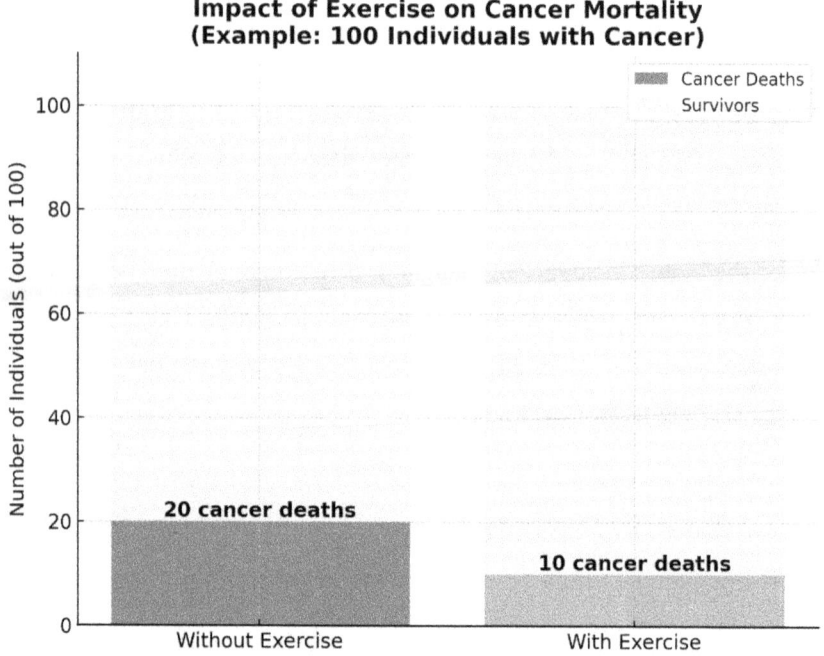

Now, you may ask: What kind of exercise provides this benefit? The answer is simple: any movement counts. Many people feel discouraged when they don't reach specific metrics, such as target heart rate zones or METs (Metabolic Equivalent Tasks). But research shows that even small doses of movement deliver significant benefits.

Take, for example, a 2023 study by Stamatakis et al. It found that just 3 to 4 minutes of brisk walking per day was associated with a 20% reduction in overall cancer risk, and a 31% reduction in risk for cancers strongly linked to physical inactivity (including breast, lung, and colon cancers).

Let that sink in: **4 minutes a day.**

Quick bursts of movement, such as taking the stairs, walking briskly through a parking lot, or hurrying between errands, can shift your health trajectory.

Even though current U.S. guidelines recommend 150 minutes per week of moderate activity, recent findings suggest that even half that amount can offer real protection. A 2023 study by Garcia et al. found that just 75 minutes per week of moderate-intensity aerobic exercise was enough to significantly lower the risk of cancer, cardiovascular disease, and overall mortality. The authors estimated that 1 in 10 premature deaths could have been prevented if everyone met this minimum threshold.

The takeaway is both simple and empowering: **it doesn't have to be perfect, it just has to begin.** Even modest amounts of activity, done consistently, can tip the scales in your favor. Your body, your cells, and your long-term health will thank you.

How Intense Should Exercise Be?

The conversation around exercise intensity is nuanced, with many variables to consider. There is strong evidence linking high levels of physical fitness to increased longevity. One noteworthy study by Mandsager et al. (2018) showed that extremely high levels of aerobic fitness were associated with the greatest reduction in long-term mortality, with particularly significant benefits observed in older adults with high blood pressure.

That said, I hesitate to recommend extreme exercise as a universal solution.

One of my favorite expressions is *Aurea mediocritas*, a Latin phrase that translates to **"the golden mean"** or **"the golden middle way."** It reflects the virtue of balance and moderation, encouraging us to avoid the extremes of both excess and deficiency.

Strenuous exercise is not without risk, particularly in individuals with underlying cardiovascular disease. Intense physical exertion raises heart rate and blood pressure, increasing **shear stress on arterial walls**. In people with soft plaques in their arteries, this stress may trigger **plaque rupture**, potentially leading to blood clots and acute cardiovascular events like heart attacks. A study by Burke et al. (1999) found that individuals who died suddenly during vigorous activity were more likely to have suffered plaque rupture compared to those who died at rest.

While regular moderate to vigorous exercise offers robust protection against heart disease, high-intensity exercise should be approached with caution, especially for those with known or suspected coronary artery disease or atherosclerosis. In such cases, pre-participation cardiovascular screening, individualized exercise prescriptions, and collaboration with a healthcare provider or cardiologist are essential for safety. In my opinion, extreme levels of exertion are not advisable for the general population.

Instead, I advocate for a more sustainable, accessible approach to movement. Below is an 8-week progressive plan designed to help someone go from complete sedentarism to consistent activity at a moderate intensity level of 5–6 METs.

Week	Goal	Type of Exercise	Duration (per session)	Frequency	Notes
1	Gentle movement	Walking (slow pace, flat surface)	10–15 min	3x/week	Focus on consistency. Avoid pain or overexertion.
2	Build habit	Walking (15–20 min), light stretching	15–20 min	3–4x/week	Add simple mobility drills or yoga.
3	Increase baseline stamina	Walking (moderate pace), bodyweight squats	20–25 min	4x/week	Introduce 5 min of uphill or faster walking.
4	Steady progress	Brisk walking (4 mph), stationary bike	25–30 min	4x/week	Aim for short intervals at a higher pace.
5	Threshold zone entry	Brisk walking + short stair climb	30–35 min	4–5x/week	Heart rate will start rising; track effort using the talk test.
6	Reach moderate intensity	Light jog (1–2 min intervals), cycling	30–40 min	5x/week	Include a dynamic warm-up and cool down.
7	Maintain & vary intensity	Swimming, dancing, elliptical	35–45 min	5x/week	Moderate intensity = breathing faster but still able to talk.
8	Consistency at 5–6 METs	Brisk walk, jog, swim, aerobics, light hike	40–50 min	5–6x/week	Use music, outdoors, or a buddy for motivation.

Activity	METs	Description
Brisk walking (4 mph)	5.0	Slightly out of breath, can talk but not sing
Leisure cycling (10–12 mph)	5.5	Flat terrain or light resistance
Light jogging	6.0	Jogging at a conversational pace
Water aerobics	5.3	Excellent for joint support and cardio
Dancing (e.g., Zumba)	5.0–6.0	Fun and energizing, helps with coordination
Elliptical (moderate)	5.0	Low-impact, full-body cardio

Tips for Success

- Warm up and cool down every session (5–10 min).
- Use the talk test: If you can talk but not sing, you're likely in the right zone.

- Track progress with a fitness watch or app (step count, heart rate, etc.).
- Listen to your body. Mild soreness is okay, while sharp pain is not.
- Hydration, recovery, and sleep are just as important as movement.

Getting from Sedentary to Moderate Exercise (5-6 METs)

Goal: Safely progress from no activity to regular moderate exercise (e.g., brisk walking, cycling, swimming)

What is 5-6 METs?

- MET = Metabolic Equivalent Task (1 MET = resting energy use)
- 5-6 METs = brisk walk, dancing, cycling at 10-12 mph

8-Week Progressive Plan:

Week 1: 10-15 min slow walk, 3x/week

Week 2: 15-20 min walk + light stretching, 3-4x/week

Week 3: 25-28 min brisker walk + bodyweight squats, 4x/week

Week 4: 25-30 min brisk walk or stationary bike, 4x/week

Week 5: 30-35 min brisk walk + stair climb, 4-5x/week

Week 6: 35-40 min light jog intervals or bike, 5x/week

Week 7: 35-45 min swim, jog, or elliptical, 5x/week

Week 8: 40-50 min at 5-6 METs, 5-6x/week

Examples of 5-6 METs Exercises:

- Brisk walking (4 mph)
- Leisure cycling (10-12 mph)
- Light jogging
- Water aerobics
- Zumba/dancing
- Moderate elliptical

Tips:

- ✓ Warm up & cool down every session
- ✓ Use the "talk test" (talking okay, singing hard)
- ✓ Stay hydrated and get good sleep
- ✓ Listen to your body – avoid overexertion

"A journey of a thousand miles begins with a single step."

In summary, exercise is one of the most powerful tools we have to protect and restore health. It improves insulin sensitivity, supports mitochondrial function, reduces inflammation, and lowers the risk of cancer, cardiovascular disease, and dementia. Whether it's a brisk daily walk, a few flights of stairs, or structured workouts, movement acts as both prevention and medicine. And perhaps most importantly, **the benefits are not all-or-nothing**; even small, consistent efforts compound over time. But while exercise lays a crucial foundation, it works best when paired with other pillars of health. In the next subchapter, we'll explore how weight management and insulin resistance further shape the trajectory of metabolic, malignant, and memory-related diseases and how this interconnectedness offers even more opportunities to intervene, repair, and thrive.

Tobacco: The One Risk Factor with No Upside

Tobacco use has declined significantly in many parts of the Western world over the past few decades, thanks to decades of public health campaigns, taxes on cigarettes, smoke-free laws, graphic warning labels, and growing cultural awareness of its harms. In the U.S., for instance, the adult smoking rate has dropped from over 40% in the 1960s to around 12% today. But globally, the story is more complex. Smoking rates remain alarmingly high in parts of Asia, including China, India, and Indonesia, where over half of the world's smokers live. In China alone, an estimated 300 million people smoke, and tobacco-related illness is projected to become one of the country's leading causes of death in the coming decades.

We've already talked in earlier chapters about the effects of smoking: it promotes **atherosclerosis, inflammation,** raises **blood pressure,** and contributes to **a long list of cancers,** especially lung cancer. And of course, we know its effect on memory and metabolism, too-both through direct vascular damage and its downstream inflammatory effects.

Despite widespread knowledge of its harms, quitting smoking is one of the most difficult behavioral changes to make. That's not a failure of willpower; it's a reflection of how powerfully addictive nicotine is, acting directly on the brain's reward system and producing withdrawal symptoms when stopped. And yet, this is one of the most impactful changes a person can make for their long-term health. That's why it's critical for physicians and healthcare providers to ask about smoking at every visit. Even if only **1 in 100** patients quits after being asked and advised to stop (Stead et al., 2013), that 1% adds up. Consistent messaging, over time, saves lives.

How to Quit: Medications, Tools, and Strategies

There are evidence-based treatments that double or triple the chances of quitting successfully. Medications and behavioral support are both important, and their combination is even more effective.

Approved Medications for Smoking Cessation:

- **Bupropion (Wellbutrin/Zyban):** An antidepressant that reduces nicotine cravings and withdrawal symptoms. It can double cessation success rates.
- **Nicotine Replacement Therapy (NRT):** Includes **patches, gum, lozenges, inhalers,** and **nasal sprays.** These help reduce withdrawal symptoms by providing controlled doses of nicotine without the harmful chemicals in cigarettes.

- **Varenicline**: A partial nicotine receptor agonist that reduces cravings and blunts the reward of smoking. It has been shown to be one of the most effective single-agent therapies.

Non-medication options:

- **Acupuncture**: Some individuals report subjective benefits, though data on long-term efficacy is limited.
- **Hypnosis**: May help certain individuals with motivation and stress management, but evidence remains inconclusive.
- **Behavioral counseling**: Individual or group therapy, even brief counseling from a clinician, increases the chance of quitting.
- **Digital tools and apps**: Text message programs and quit-smoking apps have also been shown to increase quit rates by providing daily reminders, coaching, and encouragement.

What Works Best? Comparing Methods

The following approximate **relative success rates at 6–12 months:**

Method	Quit Rate vs. Placebo
Brief physician advice	+1–3% absolute increase
Nicotine patch alone	~1.6x
Bupropion	~2.1x
Varenicline	~2.9x
Combination NRT (patch + gum/lozenge)	~2.6x
Behavioral support + meds	~3.0x

In plain terms: no single method works for everyone, but combining medication and counseling gives the best chance of success. The key is persistence, support, and trying again if the first attempt fails.

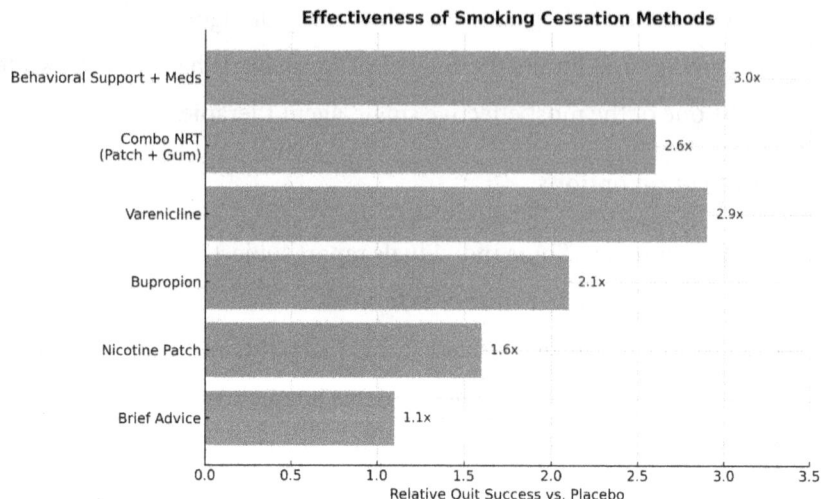

Health Recovery After Quitting

What happens after you quit? A lot of good things, some sooner than you'd think.

- **Cardiovascular risk** begins to decline within months. **After 1 year of quitting,** the risk of heart disease is cut in half. **After 5 years,** stroke risk approaches that of a non-smoker. **Within 15 years,** the risk of coronary heart disease is the same as someone who did not smoke.
- **Lung cancer death risk** decreases by **30–50% after 10 years**, and continues to decline over time, though it may never return to baseline.
- For those with emphysema or COPD, quitting smoking doesn't reverse the damage, but it slows progression dramatically, improves symptoms, and can reduce hospitalizations and flares.

Health Improvements Timeline After Quitting Smoking

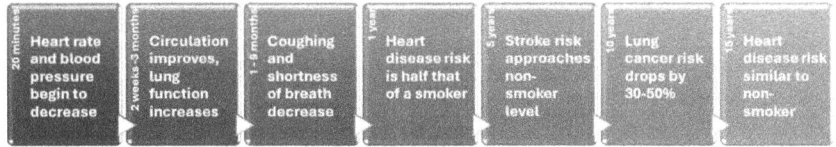

And What About Vaping?

Vaping entered the scene with bold claims of being safer than cigarettes, and while it may reduce exposure to some toxins compared to combustible tobacco, it is not risk-free. Many e-cigarettes contain high concentrations of nicotine, which can perpetuate addiction, and newer data show cardiovascular and lung effects, especially with chronic use.

As a smoking cessation aid, vaping has mixed evidence. Some studies show it can help smokers transition away from cigarettes, while others raise concern that it may prolong nicotine dependence, particularly in young users who may have never smoked before. At this point, it's not recommended as a first-line strategy for quitting smoking, and its long-term health impacts are still unfolding.

Summary

Quitting tobacco is one of the most powerful things a person can do to change their health trajectory. It's hard, but it's worth it. And we have more tools than ever before to support that journey. With persistence, the right plan, and trusted guidance, even long-time smokers can reclaim their health, one cigarette-free day at a time.

From Cigarettes to Spirits: Another Risk Worth Confronting

Just as tobacco has carved a well-documented path of harm through its effects on the heart, blood vessels, and lungs, alcohol poses its own set of threats, often underestimated and socially normalized. In the next subchapter, we'll turn our attention to alcohol: how it influences metabolic health, cancer risk, memory, and what science really says about safe use, risky thresholds, and the power of cutting back.

Alcohol: Reconsidering the "Glass of Red Wine"

Alcohol has long occupied a contradictory space in health conversations. On the one hand, it features in cultural traditions and social rituals, and even appears as an optional component in versions of the Mediterranean diet. On the other hand, mounting research continues to affirm what public health experts have cautioned for years: **no amount of alcohol is truly safe.** While small amounts of red wine are sometimes included in dietary models, such as the Mediterranean diet, these mentions are observational, not prescriptive. In other words, wine is acknowledged, not endorsed.

Let's be clear: alcohol is not a health food. It's a toxin that can exert widespread effects on multiple organ systems. Even moderate consumption has been linked to increased risks of cancer, elevated blood pressure, arrhythmias, and brain atrophy. Alcohol contributes to inflammation, impairs glucose metabolism, and can increase the risk of developing type 2 diabetes. Alcohol's impact on insulin resistance often goes unrecognized, compounding the metabolic risk.

Chronic use contributes to endothelial dysfunction, arterial stiffness, and a heightened inflammatory state, all of which feed into the M3 framework: metabolic disease, malignancy, and memory decline.

Current public health guidelines define moderate drinking as up to one drink per day for women and up to two drinks per day for men. However, this is not a recommendation to drink; rather, it **is the upper limit beyond which harm becomes increasingly likely.** Even within those limits, emerging research continues to challenge the idea that any amount of alcohol is "safe."

Despite its legal status and widespread social acceptance, alcohol is one of the most challenging substances to quit. Its deeply ingrained role in social settings ("social lubricant"), combined with its short-term mood-altering effects, makes it particularly insidious. Yet, asking patients to reduce or eliminate alcohol use during every clinical encounter is worthwhile: studies suggest that even a brief intervention can trigger a lowering of the amount of alcohol being consumed (Kaner et al, 2007).

For those ready to quit or reduce alcohol, there are several evidence-based strategies:

- Counseling & Behavioral Therapy: Cognitive Behavioral Therapy (CBT) and Motivational Interviewing have shown success in supporting long-term alcohol cessation.
- Medications:
    - Naltrexone: Blocks opioid receptors to reduce cravings and pleasure associated with alcohol
    - Acamprosate: Helps restore chemical balance in the brain disrupted by alcohol use
    - Disulfiram (Antabuse): Causes unpleasant effects when alcohol is consumed
    - Topiramate: An anti-epileptic medication that reduces cravings (used off-label)
- GLP-1 Receptor Agonists (off-label use): Although still under study, GLP-1 RAs, such as semaglutide, have shown potential in reducing alcohol intake by acting on brain reward pathways. A 2025 review by Jerlhag suggests these medications can reduce alcohol-induced reward, potentially lowering cravings and relapse risk.

Other approaches like group therapy, peer support programs (e.g., Alcoholics Anonymous), acupuncture, and even hypnosis have been explored, with varying levels of evidence. As with tobacco, success often comes from the combination of medication and counseling.

In summary, alcohol has no true health benefits and carries measurable risks even at low levels. As science continues to evolve, the public message is shifting from "drink in moderation" to "less is better, and none is best." Whether the goal is to improve metabolic health, reduce cancer risk, support cognitive function, or lower blood pressure, cutting back on or quitting alcohol is a powerful step toward undoing the damage and preventing further harm.

CHAPTER 6

How the Damage can be Undone or Prevented: Diabetes, Blood Pressure, and Cholesterol

Weight and Insulin Resistance/Diabetes

Life is beautiful, but not always fair, and this becomes especially evident when discussing weight changes over time. **As we age, gaining weight becomes easier, and losing it becomes harder.** For women, this shift often begins around the time of menopause, when declining estrogen levels lead to fat redistribution, with more fat accumulating around the abdomen and a gradual loss of muscle mass. In men, metabolic rate starts to decline in the mid-30s, driven by a slow but steady decrease in testosterone levels. This hormonal shift is typically followed by muscle loss, a slower metabolism, and a greater tendency toward fat accumulation, especially if physical activity levels also begin to drop.

As a general rule, to maintain the same weight, most individuals need to consume about 200–400 fewer calories per day in their 50s compared to what they needed at 35–40 years of age. And ideally, exercise should be stepped up, not reduced, to counterbalance the natural metabolic slowdown.

While we're on the topic of hormones, it's important to highlight that most age-related hormonal changes fall within normal physiological ranges, meaning that what's "normal" for a 50-year-old is naturally different from what's "normal" for a 20-year-old. There is no proven benefit, and real potential risks, to artificially boosting testosterone or other hormones back to youthful levels without a clear medical need. Nature adjusts these levels for a reason. There is an age-adjusted normal level that does not require overcorrection.

Coming back to the main focus of this subchapter: weight categories are typically defined using body mass index (BMI). While BMI is not a perfect measure (it doesn't differentiate between muscle and fat mass), it remains a useful and accessible tool for setting practical weight goals for the vast majority of the population.

The foundation of treating overweight and obesity is straightforward in theory: energy intake must be reduced below energy expenditure (Guyton and Hall, Textbook of Medical Physiology). In simpler terms: eat fewer calories than you burn. The National Institutes of Health (NIH) guidelines recommend reducing daily calorie intake by 500–750 kcal to achieve a weight loss of about 1 to 1.5 pounds per week. For example, this approach would result in roughly a 10% body weight loss over a six-month period for someone starting at 200 pounds. Of course, maintaining physical activity is important too, but it's worth remembering that about 80% of weight loss comes from dietary changes, not exercise alone.

The first practical step is to **calculate your daily caloric needs**. If you remember from the **Diet** subchapter, we discussed **Total Daily Energy Expenditure (TDEE)**-the combination of your **basal metabolic rate (BMR)** (your "idling" energy use) multiplied by an **activity factor (AF)** based on how much you move:

$$TDEE = BMR \times AF$$

This calculation gives us a good estimate of how many calories are needed to maintain current weight. To lose about 1–1.5 pounds per week, **a 10% reduction in TDEE** is usually a safe and effective target. (And don't worry, the DIY section of this book walks you through these calculations without the headache of formulas or a calculator needed).

But let's be honest: the math isn't the real challenge. It's easy to talk about, easy to write about, and even easy to calculate. The true difficulty lies in applying it day after day, battling against reflexes that draw us toward food, navigating a society where celebrations, holidays, and even daily rituals are centered around eating.

It's not just about knowing what to do-it's about building a system that helps us actually do it. In the DIY section, I share the practical strategies and motivation systems that have helped many of my patients and myself create reasonable, sustainable, and achievable plans for real, lasting change.

Diet-wise, there are multiple plans available, several of which we've already detailed in the **Diet** section of this book. Look carefully at their pros and cons, and ideally, choose one that includes the most "green" foods, meaning those that nourish and support healthy metabolism. However, if that doesn't feel sustainable, don't worry - choose the plan that best suits your taste, lifestyle, and rhythm. As long as you maintain a negative caloric balance, the exact dietary pattern you follow matters less than the fact that you stick with it consistently.

Understanding the process and finding ways to stay motivated are key. We know that increased weight often goes hand in hand with insulin resistance, which, over time, can lead to the development of diabetes. One of the most powerful things we can do for long-term health is to identify insulin resistance early, before it progresses to irreversible damage. That's why screening for prediabetes is so important, especially for individuals with risk factors like family history, abdominal weight gain, elevated blood pressure, or low physical activity.

The challenge is that most people don't realize they're at risk until symptoms appear or complications have already started. However, if caught early, insulin resistance presents a remarkable window of opportunity, often lasting years, during which lifestyle changes alone can halt or even reverse the trajectory.

The evidence is very clear: with modest weight loss, regular physical activity (especially a combination of aerobic exercise and strength training), and a diet low in refined carbohydrates and added sugars, many individuals with prediabetes or even early diabetes can restore normal glucose levels without needing medication.

Even in more advanced stages of diabetes, management has evolved significantly. Today, we have tools such as continuous glucose monitors, medications that protect the heart and kidneys, and a much deeper appreciation for the role of nutrition, movement, and muscle health in not just controlling the disease, but also in slowing or even partially reversing its course.

That being said, sometimes weight loss efforts plateau, or lifestyle interventions alone are not enough. And that's okay. One of the benefits of living in the 21st century is the availability of powerful, well-studied medications that can help bridge the gap.

Let's start with Metformin, a medication that has earned its reputation over decades as a safe, effective, and trustworthy option for treating both diabetes and prediabetes.

Metformin: A Foundational Tool for Metabolic Improvement

Metformin is one of the most trusted and time-tested medications in modern medicine, with over six decades of clinical use (Bailey, 2017). Most people recognize it as a go-to treatment for type 2 diabetes, but its benefits reach well beyond blood sugar control. Safe, affordable, and effective, metformin has emerged as a key ally in addressing the broader issues of metabolic health, including insulin resistance, weight gain, and inflammation—all central players in the M3 triad: metabolic disease, malignancy, and memory decline.

Why and When Metformin Is Used

Metformin is typically recommended for individuals with type 2 diabetes, especially when weight or insulin resistance are part of the picture. It's often the first medication offered at diagnosis, particularly when lifestyle changes alone haven't brought blood sugar under control. What makes metformin unique is how it works: it lowers the amount of sugar produced by the liver, increases insulin sensitivity, and helps muscles use glucose more effectively. Importantly, it achieves this without forcing the pancreas to release more insulin, which means it carries a very low risk of hypoglycemia (low blood sugar).

Metformin lowers average blood sugar (HbA1c). It's generally weight-neutral or may even promote modest weight loss, and it has favorable effects on cholesterol levels. Among oral diabetes medications, metformin is still the only one with solid, long-term evidence of reducing heart attack, stroke, and overall mortality, as demonstrated in the landmark UKPDS study (UKPDS Group, 1998).

In Prediabetes: Metformin also plays an important role before diabetes even begins. In individuals with prediabetes (those whose blood sugar is elevated but not yet in the diabetic range), it can delay or even prevent the onset of full-blown diabetes. Patel et al (2023) found that metformin reduced the risk of progressing to diabetes by 42%. While lifestyle changes show a superior benefit, metformin is a powerful second-line option when those changes aren't enough or prove difficult to maintain (Knowler 2002).

Beyond Blood Sugar: Metabolic and Weight Support

Metformin's benefits aren't limited to blood glucose. It also supports overall metabolic function by improving lipid profiles, lowering triglycerides and

LDL cholesterol, and may assist with modest weight loss in people who struggle with insulin resistance. It's frequently used in conditions like PCOS (polycystic ovary syndrome) (Lord et al, 2003) and metabolic syndrome.

When to Use Caution

Metformin is generally well-tolerated, but, like any medication, it's not suitable for everyone. Common side effects include mild gastrointestinal symptoms, such as nausea, bloating, or loose stools, which often improve over time or with a switch to an extended-release formulation. It should be used cautiously in individuals with advanced kidney disease and severe liver dysfunction. Regular kidney function monitoring is a simple and effective way to keep its use safe.

Summary

Metformin remains a cornerstone therapy for type 2 diabetes and a valuable option for those at risk due to prediabetes or metabolic dysfunction. Its ability to improve insulin sensitivity, support a healthy weight, and reduce disease progression makes it an important tool not just for managing disease, but for preventing it. As always, medication works best when paired with movement, nutrition, and a plan tailored to the individual. For many people navigating the early stages of metabolic imbalance, metformin can be a safe and effective bridge back toward better health. Additionally, a revolutionary medication, GLP-1 receptor agonists, has completely changed how we approach the treatment of Type 2 diabetes and obesity. They will be discussed in detail in the next chapter.

Blood Pressure

Blood pressure is one of the most modifiable risk factors we have. Even small, consistent improvements, through diet, exercise, weight control, stress management, and, when needed, medications, can create enormous reductions in long-term risk.

Just as we discussed earlier with blood sugar and weight, addressing blood pressure effectively is not about achieving perfection, but about understanding the tools available and moving steadily toward healthier targets. In this section, we'll explore the practical steps we can take to master blood pressure monitoring and control, undo damage, and prevent future harm.

The blood pressure recording is the starting point. While much of the discussion centers on medical office blood pressure (with patients being sent routinely to their primary care doctors or cardiologists for one value out of range in a specific medical setting), the emphasis should shift **towards home monitoring or other objective monitoring, such as a 24-hour ambulatory blood pressure monitor.**

For a blood pressure reading to be accurate, certain conditions should be met:

- The person should be sitting quietly for at least 5 minutes
- Back should be supported, feet flat on the floor
- Arm supported at heart level
- No recent caffeine, nicotine, or exercise
- No talking during the reading

The truth is, many in-office blood pressure readings don't meet these standards. They're often taken quickly, without proper positioning, sometimes right after walking in or during stressful conversations. Similarly, readings taken during emotional moments, like an argument, a medical emergency, or even at the dentist's office, may be temporarily elevated and shouldn't be the only values used to diagnose or adjust treatment.

Even those readings taken at the grocery store or pharmacy, while convenient, don't meet the accuracy standards for diagnosis or medical decisions. These machines aren't always well-calibrated, and the setting isn't controlled enough to get reliable data.

That's why there's a growing emphasis on home blood pressure monitoring. I often recommend that patients buy their own blood pressure monitor, learn how to use it correctly, and keep a log. Then, bring both the device and log to the office, so we can check that the readings match the clinic's machine (which is regularly calibrated). This helps confirm that your home readings are reproducible and reliable.

For cases where we need even more data, some clinics offer ambulatory blood pressure monitoring. This involves wearing a cuff connected to a small device (like a Walkman) that automatically checks your blood pressure every 20–30 minutes over a 24-hour period. It provides a detailed picture of how your blood pressure behaves throughout the day and night, offering a more accurate way to assess your true baseline.

The bottom line? One or two readings aren't enough. Blood pressure is dynamic, and managing it well means paying attention to patterns over time, in real-life settings, using reliable methods.

How to Check Your Blood Pressure at Home

Home monitoring is a powerful way to stay on top of your blood pressure and track trends over time. Here are the key steps to do it correctly and get reliable readings:

Choose the Right Equipment

- **Use an upper arm (arm-level) blood pressure monitor.**
  Wrist monitors are not recommended unless your arm size makes upper arm cuffs impractical. If that's the case, visit ValidateBP.org to find a validated wrist monitor.

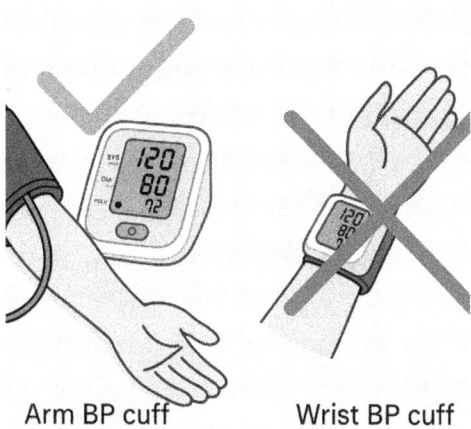

Arm BP cuff   Wrist BP cuff

- **Find a validated device.** Use ValidateBP.org to choose a trusted, clinically tested brand.
- **Measure your arm** to ensure the cuff fits properly. A poorly fitting cuff can lead to inaccurate readings.
- **Remove clothing** from your arm: always place the cuff directly on bare skin.

Prepare for an Accurate Reading

- Avoid exercise, caffeine, or smoking for at least 30 minutes before checking your blood pressure. (And yes, while we say avoid smoking before a reading, it's best to avoid it altogether.)
- Rest for at least 5 minutes before checking.
- Avoid measuring when you're feeling anxious, rushed, or emotionally stressed.
- Sit in a quiet place, back supported, feet flat on the floor, legs uncrossed. Rest your arm on a flat surface so that the middle of the cuff is at heart level.

Taking the Measurement

- Either arm is fine, but if you consistently notice higher readings on one side, use that arm from then on.
- Take your readings at the same time every day, ideally in the morning before you take any medications.
- For a more complete picture, take additional readings at different times of the day on occasion.
- Ignore the first reading-discard it completely. Wait 2 minutes, then take a second reading. Record only the second number in your blood pressure log.

How Often to Check

- Once your blood pressure is well-controlled, there's no need to check daily. A good rhythm is:
  - 2–3 times per month, ideally:
    - Once in the morning (before medication)
    - Once during the day, to capture variability
  - This keeps you engaged without causing unnecessary stress.

Bring Your Data with You

- If you've been diagnosed with high blood pressure, bring your log to every doctor's visit.
- Once a year, bring your home monitor with you to compare it to the calibrated machine at your doctor's office. If your home readings are consistently normal but your office readings run high, we typically trust the home values, but confirming that your device is accurate adds an extra layer of reassurance.

How to Check Your Blood Pressure at Home

1. Choose the Right Equipment
- Use an upper arm BP monitor
- Visit ValidateBP.org for validated devices
- Measure your arm for proper cuff fit
- Place cuff on bare skin

2. Prepare for Accurate Reading
- Avoid exercise, caffeine, or smoking 30 min before
- Rest quietly for 5 minutes
- Sit upright, back supported, feet flat
- Arm supported at heart level

3. Taking the Measurement
- Use same arm each time (whichever reads higher)
- Measure before taking medications
- Discard 1st reading, record 2nd after 2 min

4. How Often to Check
- If stable: 2-3 times per month
- Morning (before meds) and once during the day

5. Bring Your Data to Your Doctor
- Bring your BP log to every visit
- Bring your monitor yearly to compare with clinic device

6. Tips for Accurate Monitoring
- Avoid checking when stressed or ill
- Don't use wrist monitors unless absolutely necessary
- Ignore readings from pharmacy/grocery store machines

Source: Heart.org – American Heart Association

Blood Pressure Management: Lifestyle First, Medications When Needed

The first step when blood pressure is moderately elevated—something that should always be discussed with your doctor, as recommendations depend on individual health profiles—is lifestyle modification. When blood pressure is significantly elevated, medications are typically started alongside lifestyle changes.

So, what do we mean by lifestyle modifications?

- **Exercise:** Aim for at least 150 minutes of moderate-intensity activity or 75 minutes of vigorous exercise per week.
- **Stop tobacco and alcohol use:** See the dedicated subchapters for details on their impact.
- **Weight loss:** Making a sustained effort to lose weight can have a meaningful effect on blood pressure. A recent study (Yang et al., 2023) showed that blood pressure improvements are proportional to the amount of weight lost, and these benefits are even greater when combined with medical treatment.

- **Dietary changes:** Reducing salt intake plays a particularly important role. Excess dietary salt directly impacts blood pressure and cardiovascular health (He et al., 2009). A recent global call to action (Egan et al., 2025) by the World Hypertension League emphasized that reducing salt intake is an urgent and cost-effective intervention. Global estimates suggest that high sodium intake is responsible for 1.9 million cardiovascular deaths annually and contributes to roughly 7.5 million deaths from all causes. Reducing sodium intake to less than 2000 mg per day could prevent millions of deaths, much like past public health victories seen with tobacco control.

When lifestyle interventions aren't enough, medications provide a safe and highly effective way to achieve target blood pressure levels. While I won't go into the details of each medication class here—these choices are best individualized between patient and physician—it's essential to know that needing more than one medication is common and completely normal.

Rather than pushing one medication to its maximum dose, adding a second agent often provides a more balanced, multifactorial approach with greater blood pressure-lowering effects (Wald et al., 2009). Over 70% of adults treated for hypertension will require at least two medications to reach good control (Smith et al., 2020). Single-pill combination medications offer additional advantages: they improve adherence and have shown benefits in both cardiovascular outcomes and overall mortality compared to taking the same medications separately (Schmieder et al., 2023).

Fortunately, we have overwhelming safety data for blood pressure medications, regardless of the class. The benefits clearly outweigh the risks of side effects (Grossman et al., 2006), and with so many options available, medications can be adjusted or switched if side effects arise.

In short, lowering blood pressure is one of the most powerful and accessible ways to reduce cardiovascular risk, and with the right tools, it's something we can successfully address in almost everyone.

Blood Pressure Treatment and Prevention of Cardiovascular Disease and Death

A major systematic review and meta-analysis (Ettehad et al., 2016) showed that lowering systolic blood pressure by just 10 mmHg leads to remarkable reductions in risk:

- Major cardiovascular events drop by 20%
- Coronary artery disease (a key precursor to heart attacks) drops by 17%
- Stroke risk falls by 27%
- Heart failure risk decreases by 28%

In simple terms, even modest improvements in blood pressure can dramatically lower your chances of heart attacks, strokes, and hospitalizations. This isn't just about hitting a target on your blood pressure chart; it's about adding years to your life, and more importantly, adding life to those years. Put plainly: for every 10-point drop in your systolic blood pressure, you get about a 20–30% lower risk of some of the biggest health threats we face.

Another important study (Zhou et al., 2018) reinforces this message. It highlights the well-known increased risk of all-cause mortality from uncontrolled hypertension, but also brings some encouraging news: individuals whose blood pressure is treated and controlled have no significant increase in risk compared to those who never had high blood pressure to begin with. This means that treatment doesn't just slow damage; it can reverse risk. The takeaway is clear: it's never too late to intervene, and the benefits of doing so are profound.

Blood Pressure Treatment and Stroke Risk Reduction

A large review study (Lawes et al., 2004) analyzing more than 40 randomized controlled trials found that lowering systolic blood pressure by just 10 mmHg is associated with roughly a one-third reduction in stroke risk. The research clearly showed that the greater the blood pressure reduction, the greater the drop in stroke risk. Interestingly, when comparing different blood pressure medications, the study found no significant differences in their ability to reduce stroke risk, meaning it's the blood pressure control itself, not the specific drug, that matters most.

Another study (Wei et al., 2020) compared various classes of antihypertensive medications and similarly found no meaningful differences between them in reducing cardiovascular events. Across the board, the data showed a 25% reduction in cardiovascular events, a 20% reduction in cardiovascular deaths, and a 35% reduction in stroke risk. Once again, the pattern held: for every 10 mmHg drop in systolic blood pressure and every 5 mmHg drop in diastolic blood pressure, the risk of cardiovascular death, stroke, and major cardiovascular events fell significantly.

Blood Pressure Medications and Dementia

Bringing the conversation back to our M3 framework, blood pressure control plays a crucial role in protecting memory and cognitive health. A recent meta-analysis (Lennon et al., 2023), which included 17 studies and over 34,500 participants, showed that the use of blood pressure medications was associated with a significantly lower risk of developing dementia compared to individuals with untreated or uncontrolled high blood pressure. Specifically, people with uncontrolled hypertension faced up to a 42% higher risk of dementia compared to those without high blood pressure, and a 26% higher risk compared to those whose high blood pressure was effectively treated. Perhaps most encouraging, individuals with well-controlled blood pressure had no greater risk of dementia than healthy individuals without hypertension, underscoring that timely treatment can truly help level the playing field for brain health.

In summary, the evidence is overwhelming: controlling blood pressure is one of the most powerful tools we have to prevent heart attacks, strokes, kidney disease, and even memory decline. Whether through lifestyle changes, medications, or ideally both, reducing blood pressure adds not just years to life, but life to years. And importantly, it's never too late to make a difference: risk can be reduced, and in many cases, partially reversed with proper treatment.

But blood pressure is only one part of the equation. To fully address cardiovascular risk and the M3 complex of metabolic, malignancy, and memory health, we must now turn to another critical player: cholesterol.

Cholesterol

Cholesterol, specifically **LDL cholesterol**, is one of the key measurable and actionable factors we can target to improve cardiovascular health and overall well-being. For simplicity, clarity, and stronger message delivery, I focus primarily here on LDL cholesterol: the number that most directly links to heart disease risk and guides the intensity of treatment.

Yet despite being such a well-studied marker, cholesterol management is full of inefficiencies, misconceptions, and missed opportunities.

One common misconception centers on diet. I often hear, *"I eat healthy"* or *"I cook at home."* While both are admirable steps, they aren't guarantees of a heart-healthy diet. It's entirely possible to build high-calorie, high-fat meals at home, even with "healthy" ingredients. A home-cooked meal can still deliver a thousand calories or more; it's not just where you eat, but what and how much you eat that matters.

Another inefficiency occurs on the clinical side. Imagine this familiar pattern: a patient's cholesterol comes back high at their annual checkup. The doctor advises, *"Follow a healthy diet"* (perhaps Mediterranean style) and plans to recheck in three months. But nothing happens. Labs aren't repeated, diet changes may or may not have occurred, and by the next annual visit, cholesterol is still high. The cycle repeats: *"try diet, recheck labs,"* but nothing meaningful changes. It is a classic case of "kicking the can down the road," where action is postponed year after year.

A third misconception involves exercise. Don't get me wrong, exercise is wonderful, with countless benefits, but when it comes to lowering LDL cholesterol, it isn't a magic bullet. Just as exercise alone is unlikely to produce significant weight loss without dietary changes, it's also unlikely to meaningfully lower cholesterol by itself. People often enthusiastically start exercising, then feel discouraged when their cholesterol numbers barely budge. Sadly, they may abandon both exercise and cholesterol management as a result.

Lastly, let's talk about **familial hyperlipidemia.** Sometimes we see sky-high LDL cholesterol, paired with a family history of early heart attacks or very high cholesterol. We hope that diet alone will fix it. But it won't. While genetic testing for familial hyperlipidemia exists, it's not routinely performed in primary care (and not clinically indicated or recommended), and not all gene mutations are detectable. Yet the clues are often right in front of us: persistently elevated LDL, strong family history-it quacks like a duck, walks like a duck, yet we still try to believe it's something else. In these cases, delaying treatment in the hope that diet alone will correct the numbers can be dangerous.

All of this brings us to a critical tool in cholesterol management: **statins.** When lifestyle changes aren't enough, or when the cholesterol numbers, family history, or cardiovascular risk are high from the start, statins step in as one of the most well-studied and effective medications in modern medicine. In the next section, we'll explore how statins work, what they do beyond just lowering cholesterol, and why they've become a cornerstone in preventing heart attacks, strokes, and other complications tied to high LDL cholesterol.

Statins: The Foundation of Cholesterol and Cardiovascular Risk Reduction

When it comes to lowering cholesterol and reducing cardiovascular risk, statins are the cornerstone. This class of medications has been proven effective both for primary prevention (helping individuals who've never had a cardiovascular event) and secondary prevention (for those who've already experienced a heart attack, stroke, or have known coronary artery disease).

In the U.S., the statin family includes fluvastatin, lovastatin, pravastatin, simvastatin, atorvastatin, rosuvastatin, and pitavastatin. The good news: most of these medications are now available as generics, making them widely accessible and much more affordable than brand-name versions.

Each statin varies in its potency, meaning how powerfully it lowers LDL cholesterol at a given dose. Ranked by their LDL-lowering strength, the list goes roughly like this:

rosuvastatin > atorvastatin > simvastatin > pravastatin > lovastatin > fluvastatin, with pitavastatin falling somewhere between atorvastatin and simvastatin in potency.

Head-to-head studies (Jones et al., 2003) comparing statins have shown that rosuvastatin (10–40 mg) reduced LDL cholesterol by an average of 8.2% more than atorvastatin (10–80 mg), 26% more than pravastatin (10–40 mg), and 12–18% more than simvastatin (10–80 mg).

In terms of HDL cholesterol (the "good" cholesterol), rosuvastatin also led to the largest increase: +9.6% compared to +2.1% with atorvastatin and +6.8% with simvastatin at their maximum doses. While boosting HDL may not carry the same weight as lowering LDL when it comes to cardiovascular protection, it certainly doesn't hurt to have it higher.

How statins lower cholesterol, in simple terms

Statins (cholesterol-lowering medications) work by blocking an enzyme (hydroxymethylglutaryl (HMG) CoA reductase that our body uses to make cholesterol. When this enzyme is blocked, your liver cells sense that they don't have enough cholesterol inside. To fix this, the liver produces more "catchers" (called LDL receptors) that pull cholesterol out of the bloodstream and bring it into the liver for processing. As a result, the level of "bad" cholesterol (LDL) in your blood goes down.

In addition to lowering cholesterol, statins also reduce certain small building blocks (called isoprenoids) that the body uses for other cellular functions related to cholesterol production. This adds extra benefits in reducing harmful processes inside the blood vessels.

Besides decreasing LDL, most statins also have a minimal impact on raising HDL and lowering triglycerides in a dose-dependent fashion.

How do statins lower inflammation?

Although statins are best known for lowering cholesterol, they also have another important benefit: they reduce inflammation within the blood vessels. Think of cholesterol buildup (plaques) in arteries as small fires that irritate and damage the artery walls. Inflammation fuels these fires, making plaques more unstable and likely to rupture, leading to heart attacks or strokes.

Statins help by "cooling down" these fires. They lower certain chemicals in the body, known as inflammatory markers (such as C-reactive protein, or CRP), and make plaques more stable and less likely to break apart. By calming inflammation, statins not only slow plaque growth but also lower the chance of sudden problems like heart attacks.

In short, statins don't just lower cholesterol numbers; they make arteries healthier and more resilient by reducing hidden inflammation that contributes to heart disease.

Statins:
Not Just Cholesterol Pills

 Lower LDL cholesterol

 Reduce inflammation in artery walls

 Stabilize plaques to prevent rupture

 Lower risk of heart attack and stroke

Think of statins like a two-in-one treatment: they keep the pipes open and cool the fire.

Statins and Cardiovascular Risk

Statins aren't just about lowering cholesterol numbers; they're about lowering the risk of serious events and saving lives. A large meta-analysis (Lardizabal et al., 2010) that included over 70,000 patients across 25 trials found that statin therapy reduced cardiovascular events by 25% and overall mortality by 16%, regardless of the patients' starting cholesterol levels.

Even people whose LDL cholesterol was already under 100 mg/dL still benefited. This is a powerful reminder that the presence of a statin itself adds protection, even when cholesterol numbers don't seem alarming at first glance.

Another review (Singh et al., 2020), analyzing 11 trials with over 58,000 participants over a span of 26 years, showed similar impressive results: statin therapy lowered the risk of heart attack by 44% and the risk of stroke by 22%. Importantly, the study also found a reduction in all-cause mortality in high-risk patients, including individuals with diabetes. And when it comes to safety, an area many patients worry about, the study showed no significant increase in muscle pain, rhabdomyolysis (serious muscle breakdown), diabetes incidence, cancer risk, or liver problems compared to those not on statins.

Perhaps one of the most striking examples comes from the JUPITER trial (Ridker et al., 2008). This study looked at people who didn't even have high cholesterol but had elevated C-reactive protein (CRP), a marker of inflammation. Treatment with rosuvastatin reduced LDL by 50%, and the study had to be stopped early because the benefits were so strong: a 44% reduction in major cardiovascular events, 54% fewer heart attacks, 47% lower combined risk of heart attack, stroke, or death from heart disease, and a 20% reduction in death from any cause.

Taken together, these studies show that statins go beyond cholesterol control; they work on multiple levels to reduce inflammation, stabilize plaques, and protect the cardiovascular system, with benefits seen across different groups of patients, even those without obviously high cholesterol.

Statins and Dementia

Concerns about statins and memory loss frequently circulate online and in the media. Unfortunately, these worries often take hold and create a major barrier to using a medication that could otherwise offer life-saving benefits. But when we look at the actual data, the message is clear: there's no evidence that statins increase the risk of dementia. In fact, research suggests they may have protective effects for the brain.

If we return to the M3 complex of diseases introduced earlier, where inflammation is a key driver linking metabolic, malignancy, and memory decline, the benefits of statins make intuitive sense. Statins reduce inflammation, stabilize blood vessels, and improve the microvascular environment, all of which may help protect cognitive function.

A systematic review and meta-analysis of randomized trials (Ott et al., 2015) found that statin therapy did not negatively impact cognitive function, whether in individuals with normal cognition or those with Alzheimer's disease. While occasional anecdotal reports of memory changes on statins appear in clinical practice, in those rare situations, lowering the dose or switching to an alternative statin is usually sufficient to resolve the symptoms. Importantly, it's critical to maintain a strong patient-physician relationship in these cases, since fear of memory loss can easily lead someone to discontinue a medication prematurely.

In fact, rather than harming cognitive health, statins have been associated with a lower risk of dementia. A cohort study by Li et al. (2010) concluded that "statin use in early older adulthood was linked to a reduced risk of developing Alzheimer's disease." Similarly, Jick et al. (2000) found that "adults aged 50 and older who were prescribed statins had a substantially lower risk of dementia" compared to those not on the medication.

While statins are not formally part of dementia treatment guidelines, they may be a valuable part of care in patients with vascular risk factors or evidence of small vessel disease. In such individuals, statins likely provide vascular protection without harm and may even slow the progression of cognitive decline when combined with other standard dementia treatments.

Statins and Glucose Levels

It is true that statins have been associated with a **slight increase in blood sugar.** For someone already hovering near the upper end of the prediabetes range, starting a statin may push their glucose just high enough to cross into the diagnostic threshold for diabetes. But it's important to put this into perspective: this modest rise in glucose should never be a reason to avoid statin therapy.

The data is clear: the cardiovascular benefits of statins far outweigh this small risk of higher blood sugar. A large study by Ridker et al. (2012) showed that while statins slightly increase glucose, they significantly reduce the risk of heart attacks, strokes, and cardiovascular deaths. In other words, while your lab number might tip over a diagnostic line, your actual risk of life-threatening cardiovascular events is going down.

When viewed through the bigger picture of long-term health, statins remain a vital, protective therapy even for those at risk of developing diabetes.

Statins and Coronary Calcium Score: Why an Increase Isn't Bad

We have already discussed coronary calcium scoring (CAC) as a valuable tool for assessing atherosclerosis. But here is a paradox that can confuse and even discourage patients: starting a statin can lead to an increase in the coronary calcium score. At first glance, this appears to be the opposite of what we would want and can understandably lead patients to question whether the medication is effective.

However, in reality, this increase in calcium is a sign that statins are doing their job. When statins lower LDL cholesterol and reduce inflammation, they also help transform soft, unstable plaques into harder, more stable plaques. These stable plaques are less likely to rupture, the very event that triggers heart attacks and strokes. In other words, we don't mind "old, calcified plaques." We worry much more about soft, vulnerable ones that are at risk of breaking open.

A study by Ferencik et al. (2015) concluded that this plaque calcification may explain the positive clinical outcomes seen with statin therapy. Similarly, Criqui et al. (2014) found that densely calcified plaques were associated with a lower risk of cardiovascular events.

The takeaway? While it may feel counterintuitive, an increase in calcium score after starting statins is not a sign of disease worsening; rather, it indicates plaque stabilization and a lower risk of dangerous plaque rupture.

Statins and plaque regression

There is growing evidence suggesting that high-intensity statin therapy may also contribute to plaque regression, meaning a reduction in the size or volume of existing atherosclerotic plaques. This concept is particularly exciting because it implies that statins may not only prevent the progression of atherosclerosis but also reverse some of the damage.

Several clinical studies and trials have explored the potential for statins to induce plaque regression, particularly when used at high doses. Below are two key studies that provide insight into this phenomenon:

One of the landmark studies showing that statins can actually reverse plaque buildup is the ASTEROID trial (A Study To Evaluate the Effect of Rosuvastatin On Intravascular Ultrasound-Derived Coronary Atheroma Burden) (Nissen et al, 2006).

✅ **Design:** The study included 507 patients with coronary artery disease, all treated with a high-dose statin (rosuvastatin 40 mg daily) for 24 months.

✅ **Imaging:** Instead of standard imaging, researchers used intravascular ultrasound (IVUS), a highly sensitive test that can measure plaque volume directly inside the coronary arteries.

☑ **Results:**

- LDL cholesterol dropped dramatically, from 130.4 mg/dL to 60.8 mg/dL, a reduction of more than 50%.
- HDL cholesterol went up by 14.7%.
- Most importantly, plaque volume decreased by an average of 6.8% over two years.

What this means: The ASTEROID trial gave us clear, powerful evidence that intensive statin therapy doesn't just stop plaque from growing; it can make plaques shrink. It showed that lowering cholesterol aggressively doesn't just improve numbers on paper; it changes the disease inside the arteries in a meaningful way.

Another important study (Nicholls et al, 2011) published in NEJM investigated the effects of high-dose statins on plaque regression. This study compared atorvastatin 80 mg daily with rosuvastatin 40 mg daily in terms of plaque regression as measured by the percentage of the atheroma volume. This study showed that both agents induced regression of coronary artery atherosclerosis (plaque).

How Statins Shrink Plaques but Increase Calcium and Why That's a Good Thing

At first glance, it seems confusing: statins are known to slow down plaque buildup and even shrink some plaques (called plaque regression), yet they can also cause an increase in your coronary calcium score on a scan. How can both be true?

The key lies in what's happening inside the plaque. Statins help turn "soft" or "vulnerable" plaques, those that are fatty and unstable, more likely to rupture, into denser, more stable plaques. This stabilization process involves adding calcium to the plaque, acting as a protective shield, which makes it less likely to break open and cause a heart attack.

☑ **Plaque regression** means the total volume of harmful plaque is reduced.

☑ **Increased calcium score** reflects the plaque becoming denser and more stable (but still counted as "calcium" on a CT scan).

In other words, while the calcium score might go up, the plaque itself becomes less dangerous. The increase in calcium is a sign of plaque "healing" and hardening in a good way, not worsening disease.

This is one reason repeating calcium score after statin is initiated is not advisable, because statins can improve heart health even while raising calcium scores.

Statins and Liver Protection

When statins first became available, guidelines recommended frequent monitoring of liver enzymes during treatment. That was nearly three decades ago. Since then, widespread use and a growing body of research have led to an important shift: since 2012, the FDA recommends checking liver function before starting a statin, and then only if clinically indicated afterward. Simply put, routine liver monitoring is no longer required for everyone on statins, because decades of data have shown these medications are remarkably safe for the liver.

A study by Smith et al. (2003) found that only 1% of patients had liver enzyme elevations greater than three times the normal level, and 0.5% had mild elevations between two and three times the normal level. These small changes were usually linked to higher doses of statins, and in most cases, simply lowering the dose or switching to a different statin brought enzyme levels back to baseline.

Interestingly, research has uncovered another benefit: statins may actually help protect the liver. In patients with chronic liver disease, statin use has been associated with slowing disease progression, reducing the risk of liver decompensation, and even lowering mortality (Kreidieh et al., 2022). Other studies suggest statins may reduce liver fibrosis and lower the risk of liver cancer by 33% (Choi et al., 2025).

Of course, starting a statin in patients with known liver disease should be done carefully, with low doses and close monitoring of liver function. But overall, the idea that statins are inherently harmful to the liver is outdated. In fact, for many individuals, statins may offer protective effects far beyond their cholesterol-lowering role.

Statin Intolerance and the Nocebo Effect

There's no doubt that some people truly experience statin intolerance. But it's also clear that a significant portion of reported side effects may be influenced by expectations shaped by prior knowledge, whether from the internet, friends, or family. Statin intolerance is one of the clearest examples of the **nocebo effect.**

What's the **nocebo** effect? It's when someone develops side effects because they expect them to happen, even though the treatment itself isn't causing harm. The mind anticipates something negative, and the body follows.

A fascinating study by Howard et al. (2021) explored this concept. Participants received bottles of pills for a year: 4 bottles contained statins, 4 contained placebo pills, and 4 were empty (no pills). Each month, participants took the assigned bottle and recorded their symptoms.

Not surprisingly, symptoms were lowest during the months with no pills. But here's the interesting part: during the months taking statins **or** placebo pills, symptom reporting was **nearly identical, higher than in no-pill months, but there was no significant difference between the statin and placebo.** The rate of stopping the pills was also similar in both groups.

The authors concluded that **most of the symptoms attributed to statins were due to the nocebo effect.** The pattern of symptoms was the same whether participants were taking a statin or a placebo.

This study reminds us of the power of our expectations and why it's so important to have open, supportive conversations between patients and doctors.

And truly, this is the beauty of primary care medicine: an ongoing conversation, building on prior knowledge and shared understanding, where trust grows over time between patient and physician. Recognizing the nocebo effect doesn't mean dismissing symptoms; it means approaching them thoughtfully, balancing real concerns with evidence, and finding solutions together.

Statins and Muscle Damage: Understanding the Real Risks

When someone searches the internet for information on statins, muscle pain and muscle damage quickly rise to the top of concerns. It's true that statins can cause muscle-related side effects, but it's important to separate perception from reality and understand what the numbers do tell us.

The serious condition people worry about is rhabdomyolysis, which refers to muscle pain along with a measurable increase in muscle enzymes (creatine kinase, or CK) in the blood. But here is the reassuring part: rhabdomyolysis is extremely rare, occurring in about 1.5 people per 100,000 statin users. That is roughly 15 people out of a million. Or put differently: **999,985 people out of 1 million taking statins will NOT develop rhabdomyolysis.**

Muscle pain without enzyme elevation is more common, reported in 10–15% of patients, especially at higher doses. Most of the time, this discomfort is mild and goes away on its own after a few days. In other cases, doctors may lower the dose or switch to a different statin to improve tolerability.

A landmark study by Collins et al. (2016) found that muscle pain occurs in 50–100 patients out of every 10,000 statin users. The study emphasized that while muscle symptoms get a lot of attention in popular media, the actual rate of serious side effects is very low, and statins remain one of the safest, most effective, and least expensive tools for reducing cardiovascular risk.

The authors of the study make a powerful point: "While the rare cases of muscle-related side effects typically resolve quickly when the statin is stopped, the heart attacks or strokes that may occur if statin therapy is stopped unnecessarily can be devastating."

Another study (Zhang et al., 2013) showed that even in patients who stopped taking a statin due to muscle symptoms, over 90% were able to tolerate restarting the statin later, often at a lower dose or with a different formulation.

In summary, while muscle symptoms can happen, they are usually mild, manageable, and reversible. The long-term cardiovascular protection that statins provide far outweighs the small risk of muscle issues for most people.

PCSK9 Inhibitors: Another Option When Statins Aren't Enough

For individuals who truly cannot tolerate statins or who need additional LDL-lowering beyond what statins can achieve, proprotein convertase subtilisin/kexin type 9 (PCSK9) inhibitors offer a powerful alternative. These medications work by targeting a protein called **PCSK9,** which normally reduces the number of LDL receptors in the liver. By blocking PCSK9, these drugs increase the liver's ability to clear LDL cholesterol from the bloodstream, leading to significant LDL reductions.

Currently, PCSK9 inhibitors (such as **alirocumab and evolocumab**) are approved for people with familial hypercholesterolemia or established cardiovascular disease who require further LDL lowering despite statin therapy. They can be used alone or as an add-on to statins. A study by Sabatine et al. (2017) describes an LDL reduction of 59% with a PCSK9 medication. However, wider PCSK9 use has been limited by high cost, insurance barriers, and the need for injections every 2–4 weeks. Looking ahead, their role may grow as costs decrease and research expands.

A 2022 study by Khan et al. added nuance to the discussion: the researchers found that adding ezetimibe or a PCSK9 inhibitor to statin therapy lowered the risk of non-fatal heart attacks and strokes in adults at high or very high cardiovascular risk. However, this benefit wasn't seen in people at moderate or low cardiovascular risk. This finding helps guide treatment decisions, showing that these therapies have the greatest impact when targeted to the individuals at highest risk.

Ezetimibe: A Modest, Complementary Option

Ezetimibe works differently; it blocks cholesterol absorption in the gut, leading to modest reductions in LDL levels. It is often used as an add-on to statins or alone in patients who cannot tolerate statins. While safe and well-tolerated, the evidence for ezetimibe's effect on cardiovascular outcomes is less robust than for statins or PCSK9 inhibitors. Still, as the Khan study suggests, in high-risk individuals, adding ezetimibe may contribute to reduced heart attack and stroke risk.

Wrapping Up: Why Cholesterol Matters and Why to Act on It

Cholesterol is one of those rare risk factors that's **measurable, modifiable, and trackable over time.** It gives us a clear target, and with the right tools, we can hit it. Whether it is through diet, exercise, statins, or other treatments, we have solid, proven ways to lower LDL cholesterol and reduce the risk of heart attacks, strokes, and other vascular events. But managing cholesterol is not just about numbers on a lab report; it is about preserving the health of your arteries, keeping the "pipes" open, and preventing the slow, silent buildup that can lead to sudden, life-altering events.

Like many aspects of health, cholesterol control is a partnership between patient and clinician, built over time, tailored to the individual, and guided by evidence. The good news is that we do not have to wait for damage to occur before acting. The earlier we intervene, the more years of healthy life we can protect.

CHAPTER 7

GLP-1 Receptor Agonists: A Revolutionary Medication

Glucagon-like peptide-1 receptor agonists (GLP-1 RAs) have truly revolutionized the way we approach the treatment of **type 2 diabetes and obesity**. Originally developed to help manage blood sugar levels, these medications have since demonstrated powerful benefits beyond glucose control, **most notably, causing significant weight loss,** and are now being explored for a wide range of metabolic and chronic conditions.

GLP-1 RAs were first prescribed to improve glycemic control in individuals with type 2 diabetes. Over time, clinicians observed an exciting additional effect: patients consistently lost weight. This weight loss is primarily driven by two mechanisms: slowing gastric emptying (which keeps food in the stomach longer) and enhancing satiety, leading to reduced calorie intake.

Recognizing these dual benefits, pharmaceutical companies began to **develop GLP-1 RAs specifically for weight management** in addition to their role in diabetes care.

Some of the most commonly used medications in this GLP-1 RA class include:

- Ozempic© (semaglutide)
- Wegovy© (semaglutide)
- Mounjaro© (tirzepatide)
- Zepbound© (tirzepatide)
- Rybelsus© (oral semaglutide)
- Trulicity© (dulaglutide)
- Victoza© (liraglutide)

The names in parentheses are the generic names, listed here for clarity. It can be a bit confusing at first, because the same molecule-for example, semaglutide marketed under different brand names depending on whether it's intended for diabetes or weight loss.

Most newer GLP-1 RAs are administered through once-weekly injections, offering convenience for patients. Semaglutide is also available in an oral form (Rybelsus), which is taken daily, providing an alternative option for those who prefer not to use injections.

GLP-1 RA Medications: Route and Frequency

Medication	Route	Frequency
Semaglutide (Ozempic)	Injection	Weekly
Semaglutide (Wegovy)	Injection	Weekly
Semaglutide (Rybelsus)	Oral	Daily
Tirzepatide (Mounjaro)	Injection	Weekly
Tirzepatide (Zepbound)	Injection	Weekly
Liraglutide (Victoza)	Injection	Daily
Liraglutide (Saxenda)	Injection	Daily
Dulaglutide (Trulicity)	Injection	Weekly
Exenatide (Byetta)	Injection	Twice daily
Exenatide ER (Bydureon BCise)	Injection	Weekly
Lixisenatide (Adlyxin)	Injection	Daily

How GLP-1 Receptor Agonists Work

The powerful effects of GLP-1 receptor agonists in treating type 2 diabetes and obesity come from their ability to work through multiple pathways at once:

- Enhancing glucose-dependent insulin secretion: They stimulate the pancreas to release more insulin, but only when blood glucose levels are elevated, helping lower blood sugar without causing dangerous drops (symptomatic hypoglycemia).

- Suppressing glucagon release: Glucagon is a hormone that raises blood sugar. GLP-1 RAs help reduce inappropriate glucagon levels, improving overall glucose balance.
- Slowing gastric emptying: By delaying how quickly the stomach empties, they promote longer satiety and more gradual glucose absorption, both of which help stabilize blood sugar levels.
- Acting on the central nervous system: GLP-1 RAs influence brain pathways that regulate appetite and fullness, helping people feel satisfied with smaller meals.
- Modulating hunger hormones like ghrelin: They help decrease the sensation of hunger by lowering levels of ghrelin, often referred to as the "hunger hormone."

These combined effects are what make GLP-1 receptor agonists so effective: they not only improve blood sugar control but also support meaningful weight loss, offering a dual benefit for individuals navigating type 2 diabetes and obesity.

GLP-1 Receptor Agonists and Mitochondrial Health

Is there a connection between GLP-1 receptor agonists and mitochondrial function? The answer is yes, and it's an exciting part of how these medications deliver benefits beyond just blood sugar and weight loss.

GLP-1 RAs have been shown to improve mitochondrial efficiency and reduce oxidative stress, key factors in slowing the progression of metabolic diseases. A study by Luna-Marco et al. (2023) demonstrated that GLP-1 RAs can enhance mitochondrial performance while lowering harmful inflammation and oxidative damage. In addition, these medications improve inflammatory markers and reduce white blood cell interactions with arterial walls, both early steps in the development of atherosclerosis (see also the chapter *How Damage Is Done*).

They even go a step further: GLP-1 RAs have been found to reduce **carotid intima-media thickness (CIMT)**, a marker of early atherosclerosis.

What is CIMT? It's a non-invasive ultrasound measurement of the two inner layers (intima and media) of the carotid arteries, which supply blood to the brain. Increased CIMT reflects early plaque buildup and vascular aging. Reducing CIMT is associated with a lower risk of future cardiovascular events.

Further supporting evidence comes from studies like Wang et al. (2023), which showed improved mitochondrial function at the kidney level in animal models, helping explain why GLP-1 RAs protect kidney health. Similarly, at the heart level, GLP-1 RAs were shown to diminish oxidative stress in cardiac mitochondria (Nuamnaichati et al., 2020), supporting their cardioprotective effects.

In summary: GLP-1 receptor agonists positively influence mitochondria by enhancing energy production, reducing oxidative stress, promoting the removal of damaged mitochondria, and improving how cells use nutrients. These cellular improvements help explain the wide-ranging benefits they offer in conditions such as type 2 diabetes, diabetic nephropathy, and cardiovascular disease.

I realize that diving into mitochondrial mechanisms might feel like getting into the weeds. But understanding the basics of how these medications work at the cellular level builds confidence, deepens patient engagement, and creates a more meaningful connection to the therapeutic journey.

And now, let's shift our focus back to the clinical impact, which is the real-world benefit we see in patients every day, supported by the best available medical literature.

GLP-1 Receptor Agonists: Impact on Type 2 Diabetes

The initial indication for GLP-1 receptor agonists (GLP-1 RAs) was the treatment of type 2 diabetes. These medications have been available for many years, but earlier formulations had a less pronounced effect on weight, which initially limited their popularity. Their use has expanded dramatically as the powerful weight loss effects have become better understood; yet, their primary role in managing blood glucose in type 2 diabetes remains well established.

In type 2 diabetes, GLP-1 RAs are commonly used alone or in combination with other agents such as metformin and/or insulin. They are not typically used for glucose control in type 1 diabetes.

The choice of which GLP-1 RA to prescribe often depends on the individual's other health conditions, such as cardiovascular disease, sleep apnea, fatty liver disease, or kidney disease, since some agents have specific added benefits. However, choosing between different GLP-1 RAs based on these factors is beyond the scope of this book.

In terms of measurable outcomes, one of the primary ways we track diabetes control is through Hemoglobin A1c, which measures the average blood glucose level over the past 2–3 months.

A review of multiple randomized clinical trials by Htike et al. (2017) showed that GLP-1 RAs consistently improve glucose control (as measured by reductions in Hemoglobin A1c) and promote weight loss. The review also noted that gastrointestinal symptoms, especially nausea and vomiting, were more common compared to placebo, though these side effects are typically dose-related and often improve with time.

More recently, a meta-analysis published in 2024 by Yao et al. confirmed these findings: GLP-1 RAs significantly improved blood glucose control and supported meaningful weight loss across a variety of patient populations.

GLP-1 Receptor Agonists and Weight Loss

The impact of GLP-1 receptor agonists on weight loss is no longer just something discussed in medical journals; it's a phenomenon many of us see unfolding in everyday life. Even without a background in medicine, we hear stories in the media, see testimonials from public figures, or notice friends and family members who have experienced significant weight loss with these medications.

A recent review by Qin et al. (2024) analyzed seven randomized controlled trials involving over 4,500 individuals and concluded that once-weekly tirzepatide led to remarkable and sustained weight loss, with a favorable safety and tolerability profile. Interestingly, the degree of weight loss was dose-dependent:

- **5 mg dose**: 8.07% weight loss (approximately 7.5 kg = 16.5 lbs)
- **10 mg dose**: 10.79% weight loss (approximately 11.0 kg = 24 lbs)
- **15 mg dose**: 11.83% weight loss (approximately 11.5 kg = 25 lbs)

Another important study by Rodriguez et al. (2024) compared two of the most widely used GLP-1 RA medications, semaglutide and tirzepatide. Their findings showed that patients on tirzepatide lost more weight than those on semaglutide, with an average difference of 6.9% greater weight loss at the 12-month mark.

Importantly, adverse effects were similar between the two groups, reinforcing the overall safety profile of these medications.

GLP-1 Receptor Agonists and Blood Pressure

In addition to improving blood sugar and promoting weight loss, GLP-1 receptor agonists also have a beneficial effect on blood pressure. The same review by Qin et al. (2024) mentioned earlier noted a dose-dependent decrease in both systolic and diastolic blood pressure among individuals treated with tirzepatide.

Tirzepatide dose	5 mg	10 mg	15 mg
Systolic BP	-4.86 mmHg	-5.3 mmHg	-6.4 mmHg
Diastolic BP	-1.9 mmHg	-2.25 mmHg	-2.86 mmHg

Further supporting this, a randomized controlled trial by Lincoff et al. (2023) showed that over a 40-month period, patients taking semaglutide had a 5.1 mm Hg lower systolic blood pressure compared to those receiving a placebo.

While it's commonly expected that weight loss leads to lower blood pressure, and that certainly plays a role, these studies suggest there's more to the story. The blood pressure reduction appears to have components independent of weight loss, pointing to direct vascular or hormonal effects from the medication itself.

This adds yet another layer of benefit to GLP-1 RAs, reinforcing their growing role not just in metabolic health but in overall cardiovascular protection as well.

GLP-1 Receptor Agonists and Cardiovascular Benefits

Beyond their impact on blood sugar and weight, GLP-1 receptor agonists have shown remarkable cardiovascular benefits.

A meta-analysis by Qin et al. (2022), which included six randomized controlled trials and over 52,000 patients with type 2 diabetes, found that GLP-1 RA therapy reduced the risk of death from cardiovascular causes by 10% and lowered the risk of fatal or non-fatal stroke by 15% compared to placebo.

Similarly, another analysis by Giugliano et al. (2021) confirmed that GLP-1 RAs decrease major adverse cardiovascular events (MACE), including stroke, heart attack, and cardiovascular death, while also reducing hospitalizations for heart failure and lowering all-cause mortality.

Excitingly, these benefits are not limited to patients with diabetes.

A randomized trial by Lincoff et al. (2023) studied overweight and obese individuals with cardiovascular disease but without diabetes. Over approximately 3.5 years, the GLP-1 RA semaglutide reduced the incidence of major adverse cardiovascular events by 20% compared to placebo.

Importantly, this benefit was not solely attributed to weight loss (although patients did lose about 9.4% of their body weight at 2 years), but also to a reduction in systemic inflammation, a key driver of cardiovascular disease. Moreover, the benefits appear relatively early during treatment.

A study by Kosiborod et al. (2023) in patients with heart failure showed that, after just one year, patients receiving GLP-1 RA therapy experienced improved exercise capacity, significant weight reduction (~13.3%), decreased inflammatory markers, and an overall improvement in quality of life.

GLP-1 Receptor Agonists and Sleep Apnea

Another exciting development in the field of metabolic health is the emerging role of GLP-1 receptor agonists in treating sleep apnea. In 2024, the U.S. Food and Drug Administration (FDA) approved tirzepatide for the treatment of obstructive sleep apnea, marking a major milestone in expanding the therapeutic uses of this class.

Supporting this, a recent study by Li et al. (2025) demonstrated that GLP-1 RA therapy significantly reduced symptoms of sleep apnea. Patients not only experienced improved breathing patterns during sleep but also saw accompanying benefits, including reductions in blood pressure and meaningful weight loss.

This recognition reinforces the idea that GLP-1 receptor agonists are not just glucose or weight medications; they are reshaping the management of multiple chronic diseases rooted in metabolic dysfunction.

GLP-1 Receptor Agonists and Fatty Liver Disease

Fatty liver disease is a common but often overlooked condition that, if left untreated, can progress to liver cirrhosis, end-stage liver disease/liver failure. Given the close relationship between obesity, insulin resistance, and fatty liver, it's intuitive to expect that weight loss would improve liver health, and thankfully, the data strongly supports this.

A study published in the New England Journal of Medicine by Loomba et al. (2024) demonstrated that tirzepatide leads to dose-dependent improvements in fatty liver changes, offering significant hope for patients at risk. Additionally, a systematic review by Potter et al. (2025) concluded that treatment with GLP-1 receptor agonists in individuals with fatty liver disease likely results in improvement seen on both liver biopsy and imaging studies.

GLP-1 receptor agonists are emerging as valuable tools for liver health, reducing liver fat, helping to resolve fatty liver (the new medical term is MAFLD = Metabolic Dysfunction-Associated Fatty Liver Disease), and slowing fibrosis progression.

By addressing both metabolic dysfunction and inflammation at the root, they are reshaping the treatment of this chronic liver disease.

GLP-1 Receptor Agonists and Kidney Benefits

Another important and often underappreciated benefit of GLP-1 receptor agonists is their positive impact on kidney health. The study by Giugliano et al. (2022) showed a significant reduction in the amount of protein in urine, an important early marker of diabetic kidney disease progression. Lowering urinary protein (albuminuria) is crucial because it signals less ongoing kidney damage.

More recently, a landmark trial led by Perkovic et al. (2024) highlighted the benefits of semaglutide for patients with type 2 diabetes and moderate to severe chronic kidney disease. In this study, semaglutide slowed the progression of kidney disease, leading to a 24% reduction in major kidney outcomes (such as kidney failure and kidney-cardiovascular death) compared to placebo.

Even more impressive, semaglutide reduced death from cardiovascular causes by 29% and lowered all-cause mortality by 20%. Participants also experienced a slower decline in kidney function and had fewer serious adverse events, emphasizing not just efficacy but also safety. This trial reinforces the idea that GLP-1 RAs offer dual benefits: improving glycemic control while protecting kidney function, and along the way, reducing cardiovascular events and saving lives in patients at highest risk.

GLP-1 Receptor Agonists and Cancer Risk Reduction

As discussed earlier in the chapter *How the Damage Is Done*, increased weight is associated with a higher risk of developing certain types of cancer. Interestingly, GLP-1 receptor agonists appear to counteract some of that risk, offering yet another powerful benefit beyond glucose control and weight management.

A large retrospective study by Wang et al. (2024), involving over 1.6 million patients with type 2 diabetes, found that those treated with GLP-1 RAs had a significantly lower risk of developing 10 out of 13 studied cancers compared with patients treated with insulin.

The cancers with notable risk reduction included:

- Gallbladder cancer
- Meningioma
- Pancreatic cancer
- Hepatocellular carcinoma
- Ovarian cancer
- Colorectal cancer
- Multiple myeloma
- Esophageal cancer
- Endometrial cancer
- Kidney cancer

Another study suggested that GLP-1 RA therapy may also reduce the risk of developing hematologic cancers. Although a direct causal link hasn't been definitively proven, the association is consistent with findings from other studies.

Importantly, the reduced cancer risk appeared to be independent of glucose control, suggesting that the benefits may stem from lower systemic inflammation, a known driver in the development of conditions such as myelodysplastic syndrome and other myeloproliferative neoplasms.

Further supporting this, a large cohort study by Levy et al. (2024), which included over 1.1 million patients, found that GLP-1 RAs, particularly semaglutide, were associated with a reduced risk of several major cancer types.

The study noted lower incidences of gastrointestinal, skin, breast, female genital, prostate, and hematologic cancers among those treated with GLP-1 RAs, with semaglutide showing the strongest protective effect, particularly against gastrointestinal cancers.

GLP-1 Receptor Agonists and All-Cause Mortality

At this point, it may start to sound too good to be true, but the data supporting GLP-1 receptor agonists remains overwhelmingly positive. And importantly, it's true, backed by high-quality studies.

A major analysis published in The Lancet by Sattar et al. (2021) looked at eight randomized controlled trials (RCTs)-considered the gold standard in medical research-covering over 60,000 individuals.

The findings were remarkable:

- GLP-1 RA therapy **reduced all-cause mortality by 12%.**
- **Major adverse cardiovascular events (MACE) were reduced by 14%.**
- Hospital admissions for heart failure dropped by 11%.
- Composite kidney outcomes improved by 21%.

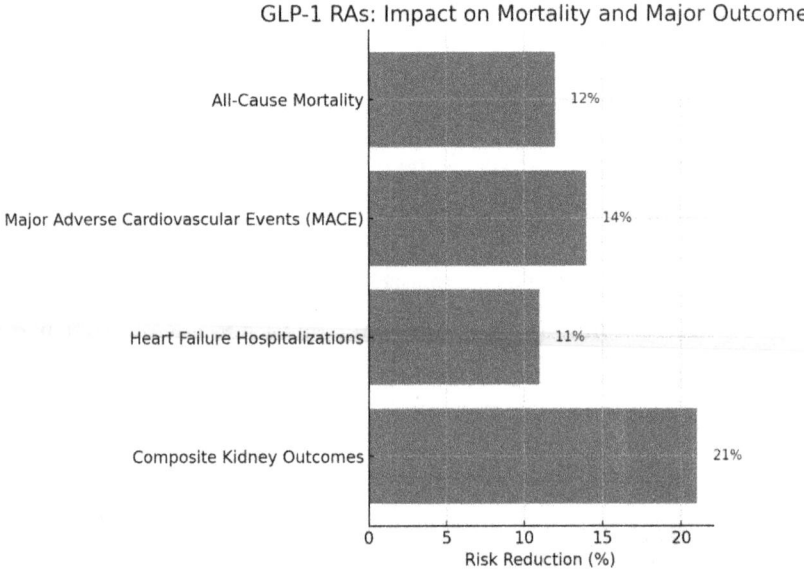

Adding to this, a retrospective cohort study including over 140,000 patients found that tirzepatide, a newer medication in the GLP-1 RA family, was associated with even greater reductions in all-cause mortality and a lower risk of diabetic kidney disease compared to other GLP-1 RA medications.

What makes tirzepatide unique is its dual mechanism: Besides acting as a GLP-1 receptor agonist, it also has GIP receptor agonist (GIP-RA) properties. GIP (glucose-dependent insulinotropic polypeptide) is a hormone released after eating that stimulates insulin secretion. In many individuals with diabetes, the GIP response is blunted; tirzepatide helps restore this, offering synergistic metabolic benefits through a two-pronged approach.

GLP-1 Receptor Agonists and Alcohol Use

GLP-1 receptors in the brain are closely connected to our reward pathways, the system that helps us experience pleasure and shapes motivation. When we engage in an enjoyable activity, like eating a favorite meal, the brain releases **dopamine**, often called the "feel-good" chemical. Dopamine reinforces pleasure by creating neural circuits that signal to the brain, *"That felt good, let's do it again."* But in today's world, with constant exposure to highly stimulating rewards, whether it's processed foods, social media, alcohol, gambling, or addictive substances like nicotine, we've set the stage for trouble. Over time, the brain begins to crave larger hits of dopamine just to achieve the same level of satisfaction, setting the groundwork for overuse, dependence, or addiction.

This may help explain the intriguing connection between GLP-1 receptor agonists and reduced substance use. Brunchman et al. (2019) conducted a systematic review of rodent studies and found that GLP-1 RAs showed inhibitory effects on substance use disorders, including nicotine, alcohol, and other drugs. More recently, Jerlhag (2025) reported that preclinical studies demonstrate that "GLP-1 RAs decrease alcohol intake, reduce motivation to consume alcohol, and prevent relapse drinking by potentially lowering alcohol-induced reward".

Although human studies are still underway, I've observed in my own clinical practice that some patients on GLP-1 RAs report decreased alcohol consumption. While these are anecdotal observations, they highlight the exciting possibility that GLP-1 RAs may one day play a role in treating not only substance use disorders but potentially other compulsive behaviors such as gambling or social media overuse. Robust research is needed, but the potential is promising.

Precautions When Starting GLP-1 Receptor Agonists

Before initiating GLP-1 receptor agonist therapy, there are a few important safety considerations to review. One of the most common questions relates to any personal or family history of medullary thyroid cancer or multiple endocrine neoplasia (MEN) syndrome types 2A or 2B, both rare, but important conditions involving hormone-secreting tumors.

Fortunately, medullary thyroid cancer is quite rare, accounting for only 1–2% of all thyroid cancers in the United States. The vast majority of thyroid cancers are papillary thyroid cancer (about 70–85%) or follicular thyroid cancer (about 10–15%).

It's important to note that GLP-1 RAs are contraindicated in patients with a personal or family history of medullary thyroid cancer or MEN 2A/2B syndromes.

They are not contraindicated in individuals with a personal or family history of other thyroid cancers, such as papillary or follicular thyroid cancer.

Adding further reassurance, a large cohort study by Pasternak et al. (2024), which included over 145,000 patients across Denmark, Norway, and Sweden, found that GLP-1 RA treatment was not associated with a substantial increase in the risk of thyroid cancer.

Another concern sometimes raised is the risk of pancreatitis. While caution is advised if someone has a history of pancreatitis, the current evidence is reassuring:

A recent study by Ayoub et al. (2025) concluded that the use of GLP-1 RAs did not increase the risk of pancreatitis; in fact, it was associated with a lower rate of pancreatitis compared to patients not treated with GLP-1 RAs.

Another safety highlight:

A study by Huang et al. (2024) found that GLP-1 RA therapy was associated with a lower risk of acute kidney injury and allergic reactions, adding to their already favorable safety profile.

One important point to remember when using GLP-1 receptor agonists is that the weight loss achieved is not limited to fat mass: lean muscle mass can be lost as well.

Preserving muscle is crucial, especially for maintaining long-term metabolic health, mobility, and strength as we age. Because overall calorie intake often decreases with these medications, it's essential to counsel patients on the importance of a nutrient-dense, high-protein diet.

Prioritizing foods rich in protein, both plant-based and animal-based sources, can help protect and rebuild muscle even as weight decreases. Simple strategies, such as adding legumes, nuts, seeds, tofu, eggs, fish, or lean meats, can make a big difference in preserving muscle during weight loss.

In parallel, building and maintaining muscle through exercise is equally important. Incorporating strength-focused activities, such as resistance training, weightlifting, or body-weight exercises (like squats, lunges, and push-ups), should become a cornerstone of the lifestyle plan whenever possible.

This combination, smart nutrition and intentional movement, ensures that the weight lost is a healthier weight and that the metabolic gains achieved through GLP-1 RA therapy are maximized and sustainable.

As with any new medication, close clinical follow-up and careful observation for potential side effects are essential.

Gradual dose titration, slowly increasing the medication dose to the target level, is key to minimizing gastrointestinal side effects such as nausea, vomiting, or constipation.

In my personal clinical experience over the past several years, GLP-1 RAs have been generally very well tolerated, and the rate of discontinuation is low when titration is done thoughtfully and patients are guided to adjust portion sizes as needed.

Barring any unforeseen future reports of concerning side effects, GLP-1 receptor agonists appear to be an overall safe and robust therapeutic class.

With ongoing positive studies highlighting multisystemic benefits across cardiovascular, renal, metabolic, and even cancer outcomes, this is a class that has stood the test of time.

It's hard to believe that nearly two decades have passed since the first GLP-1 RA, exenatide, was approved for diabetes treatment in 2005, a testament to its proven safety and the expanding horizon of benefits it continues to offer.

GLP-1 Receptor Agonists Treatment Cost

The potential of GLP-1 receptor agonists to change the trajectory of chronic diseases is enormous, yet access remains a major barrier. Despite the proven benefits for patients with type 2 diabetes, obesity, cardiovascular disease, and even emerging benefits in sleep apnea and fatty liver disease, many individuals in the U.S. cannot afford these medications. Significant insurance hurdles persist even for patients with clear indications like diabetes, with coverage often restricted, denied, or burdened by layers of prior authorizations. For newer or secondary indications, such as weight loss, sleep apnea or metabolic liver dysfunction, the situation is even more challenging, leaving many patients unable to access therapy unless they turn to compounded alternatives. Unfortunately, compounded products can vary in quality, availability, and regulatory approval, creating uncertainty and gaps in care.

In response, some manufacturers have developed their own pharmacy systems, allowing physicians to prescribe directly, with medications shipped to patients on a cash-pay basis, but at a steep cost, often between $350–550 per month. While this is less expensive than traditional retail prices, it remains unattainable for many.

One would hope that the demonstrated benefits, including reductions in all-cause mortality, hospitalizations, and disease complications, would eventually translate into economic incentives for insurers to expand coverage, recognizing that investing in prevention pays long-term dividends in both human and financial terms. Improving access to GLP-1 RAs is not just about treating disease; it's about shifting the health trajectory of entire populations toward longer, healthier lives.

Economically, the widespread adoption of GLP-1 RAs will likely disrupt multiple industries. Healthcare spending patterns could shift dramatically, with lower costs in areas like cardiovascular interventions, cancer treatment, and hospital admissions. At the same time, industries reliant on chronic disease maintenance, ranging from dialysis centers to bariatric surgery providers, may face significant transformation in the coming years.

In summary, weight management is one of the most powerful levers available for improving metabolic health, reducing insulin resistance, and preventing or even reversing early-stage diabetes. We've explored how lifestyle changes, particularly around diet, movement, and mindset, remain the foundation of success, while medications like metformin and GLP-1 receptor agonists offer additional tools when lifestyle alone isn't enough. Addressing weight isn't about chasing a number on the scale-it's about restoring the body's balance, improving resilience, and lowering the risk of many downstream diseases across the M3 spectrum.

But weight is only one piece of the puzzle of health maintenance.

CHAPTER 8

Health Maintenance

After exploring how the damage is done and how much of it can be undone, it's time to talk about what we can do to stay ahead of disease in the first place. That's where health maintenance comes in. It's the quiet, consistent work of prevention: keeping tabs on our numbers, catching problems early, and reducing risk before symptoms ever show up. While treatments and reversals are possible, nothing beats staying in the clear to begin with. This chapter focuses on the pillars of proactive health: understanding what health maintenance really means, staying up to date with screenings and immunizations, working closely with your primary care provider, and tracking vital indicators like blood pressure, blood sugar, and cholesterol. The goal is simple-more healthy years, fewer surprises.

What is Health Maintenance?

Health maintenance is the part of medical care that focuses not on treating illness, but on staying well, on protecting what's working, catching what isn't working at an early stage, and guiding people toward choices that help them thrive. At its core, health maintenance is about prevention: identifying diseases before symptoms appear, preventing illnesses when possible (through tools like immunizations), and managing known conditions to keep them under control. It also includes something that's often overlooked: empowering people with information about diet, exercise, sleep, stress, and other aspects of daily life that deeply affect our health and well-being.

The goal is to maintain an optimal state of health for as long as possible.

Health maintenance begins before we are born. It starts with prenatal screening for genetic or developmental conditions and continues throughout every phase of life. Recommendations differ based on age, sex, risk factors, and personal health history, and they evolve over time as science uncovers new evidence. What we recommend today may not be exactly what we recommend ten years from now, and that's a good thing. It means we're learning, adjusting, and getting better at helping people live longer, healthier lives.

Traditionally, health maintenance includes elements like cancer screenings, cholesterol checks, blood pressure monitoring, diabetes screening, vaccinations, and counseling on smoking cessation or alcohol use. But I'd like to widen the lens a bit. Sleep, although not always listed as part of formal health maintenance, is a pillar of physical and mental health. Poor sleep is tied to everything from heart disease to depression to impaired memory and immune dysfunction. So, in this book, I've chosen to treat it as an essential component of health maintenance.

Health maintenance isn't just a checklist; it's a philosophy. It is the idea that your health is worth guarding, even when nothing feels wrong. It is a commitment to consistency over crisis, to nurturing resilience rather than waiting for breakdowns. And it's deeply personal. What's right for one person at 25 may be very different at 55, 75, or beyond. That's why working with a trusted primary care team is so important: they help tailor recommendations to your life, your risks, and your goals.

In the sections ahead, we'll break down the major parts of health maintenance: cancer screening, immunizations, the role of the primary care physician, sleep, and more.

But remember, this isn't just about following rules; it's about creating a lifestyle where your body and mind are supported year after year. Prevention isn't flashy, but it works, and it's one of the most powerful tools we have.

Screening for Cancer

Let's start with the basics: what is cancer screening? In the simplest terms, screening is the process of looking for disease before symptoms appear. It's not diagnosis, and it's not treatment; it's the search for hidden illness in people who feel perfectly fine. The idea is to catch certain cancers early, when they are most treatable, and sometimes even curable.

But not every cancer qualifies for screening. We don't screen for every disease under the sun; we only screen for those that meet certain criteria. First, a particular cancer must occur often enough in the population to justify screening. Second, there must be a good, safe test available that can detect the disease early enough to make a meaningful difference. And third, most importantly, there must be a "window" of opportunity—a time when the cancer is present but hasn't yet caused harm—and catching it in that window improves outcomes.

To bring this concept to life, let me share a metaphor I came across called "the barnyard analogy." I wish I knew who first came up with it, but it's such a powerful visual that it deserves a place here anyway.

Imagine a barnyard with three animals inside: a turtle, a rabbit, and a bird. The goal is to keep them inside the barn. The turtle moves so slowly that even if the door is left open for a while, it's unlikely to wander far. The rabbit, however, will dart out the door if it's left open for just a bit too long; you have to be quick and catch it in time. The bird? It flies away the moment the door cracks open; there is no chance of keeping it in.

This is cancer screening in a nutshell. Some cancers are turtles; they grow so slowly that even if we don't catch them, they may never cause harm in a person's lifetime. Others are birds, so aggressive and fast-moving that even regular screening might miss them entirely, or they show up between screenings. But the cancers we aim to catch with screening are the rabbits;

they move fast enough to matter, but slow enough that we still have a real chance to catch them early and act.

That's why screening guidelines focus on certain cancers like breast, colon, cervical, and lung cancer in high-risk individuals. These are our "rabbits": common enough to warrant attention, and beatable when found early. For instance, colonoscopies can catch and even remove precancerous polyps before they ever become cancerous. Mammograms help identify breast tumors before they can be felt. Pap smears and HPV testing can spot early changes in cervical cells before cancer develops. And low-dose CT scans for high-risk individuals can identify lung cancer in a stage when surgery might still be curative.

It's important to understand that no screening test is perfect. There can be false positives, false negatives, and sometimes findings that cause stress but turn out to be harmless. But when thoughtfully applied, cancer screening saves lives, not by preventing disease from ever appearing, but by giving us a fighting chance to catch it early and respond wisely.

Cervical Cancer Screening

Cervical cancer is one of the most preventable forms of cancer, and that's thanks in large part to effective screening tools. The cervix is the lower, narrow part of the uterus that connects to the vagina. It plays an important role in reproductive health, but it's also a site where cancer can develop over time, often silently and slowly. That's where the screening comes in.

There are several ways to screen for cervical cancer, and the most well-known is the Pap smear. This test involves gently swabbing the surface of the cervix to collect cells, which are then sent to a laboratory for analysis. There, a pathology expert examines them under a microscope to look for any abnormal or precancerous changes. The goal is to identify any issues before they progress into something more serious.

Pap smears can be done with or without a test for HPV (human papillomavirus), a common virus that plays a key role in most cases of cervical cancer. There are many strains of HPV, and while most are harmless and go away on their own, a few high-risk types can lead to cancer if left unchecked. That's why testing for HPV alongside the Pap smear (called co-testing) or testing for HPV alone has become an important part of screening. It helps doctors assess the true risk and tailor follow-up accordingly.

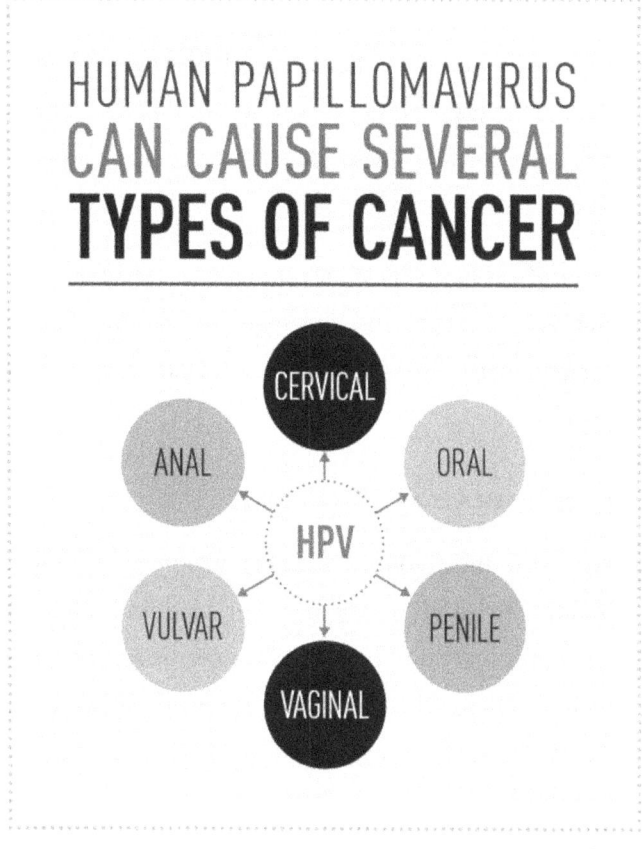

Image: The human papillomavirus (HPV) can cause several types of cancer. For example, almost all cases of cervical cancer are caused by HPV. HPV vaccination has the potential to reduce cervical cancer incidences around the world by two-thirds.

Source: National Cancer Institute (NCI)

HPV testing can even be done at home, using a self-swab that's mailed to a lab. This option can make screening more accessible and comfortable for many people, especially those who feel hesitant or anxious about in-office exams. And expanding access matters, because the more people we screen, the more lives we save.

Screening typically begins at age 21 and continues until about age 65, but the exact timing and type of test may vary. Some people may need to continue beyond age 65, especially if they've had abnormal results in the past or other risk factors like a history of HPV or a weakened immune system. That's why it's always important to discuss your individual situation with your doctor. These guidelines provide a foundation, but personalized care is key.

The real power of cervical cancer screening is in catching changes early, when they are easily treatable and long before cancer ever has a chance to develop. Like with many things in health maintenance, the earlier we look, the better we do.

Screening for Breast Cancer in Women

Breast cancer is the most common cancer diagnosed in women in the United States and the leading cause of cancer death in women worldwide. In the U.S., it ranks second only to lung cancer in cancer-related deaths among women. But here's the good news: the rate of breast cancer deaths in the U.S. has declined significantly over the past few decades. One of the biggest reasons for this progress is screening.

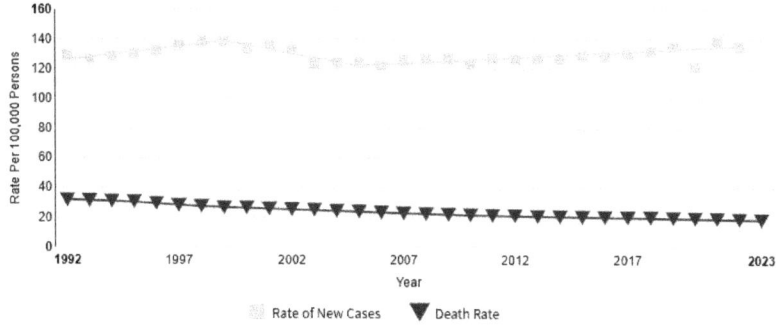

Image: *Female breast cancer new cases (126 per 100,000 in 1992 to 135 per 100,000 in 2023) and death rate (decreased from 32.1 to 18.7 per 100,000 from 1992 to 2023 in the US). Source: National Cancer Institute (NCI)*

Breast cancer screening allows us to detect cancer early, often before symptoms develop and while treatment is most likely to succeed. The primary tool for screening is the mammogram, an X-ray of the breast that can reveal small tumors long before they can be felt. For women of average risk, screening mammography typically begins at age 40, although this may vary depending on medical history, personal preference, or updated guidelines. Some women may be advised to start earlier, particularly those with a strong family history of breast cancer, a known genetic mutation (like BRCA1 or BRCA2), or a personal history of radiation to the chest.

Sometimes, breast ultrasound may be added to the screening process, especially for women with extremely dense breasts, where mammograms may not show the tissue as clearly. But ultrasound alone is not recommended as a primary screening tool. For women at very high risk, such as those with a calculated lifetime risk of breast cancer greater than 20%, breast MRI is often used in addition to mammograms to improve detection.

It's important to make a clear distinction here between screening and diagnostic imaging. Screening applies to people who have no symptoms; no lumps, no breast discharge, and no skin changes. The goal is to catch cancer before it causes problems. However, once a lump or other abnormality is discovered, whether by a doctor or during a self-exam, the situation changes. At that point, you are no longer in the screening zone; you are in the diagnostic zone. And that's when additional tests, such as a diagnostic mammogram, targeted ultrasound, or breast MRI are tailored to evaluate what's been found.

Some people also ask about clinical breast exams; that is, having a clinician physically examine the breasts as part of a routine checkup. While this was once part of screening guidelines, it's no longer recommended as a primary screening tool. That said, it still plays an important role in evaluating a specific concern, like a palpable lump or skin change.

When it comes to how often to screen, guidelines suggest every 1–2 years, depending on age and risk. In my own practice, I lean toward annual screening, particularly between the ages of 40 and 75. I choose this approach because I had breast cancer diagnosed at 1 year or so from a prior normal mammogram in my clinical practice, so I prefer to err on the side of caution.

When to stop breast cancer screening is a more nuanced discussion. Unlike cervical cancer, where prior normal results and age can help define a clear stopping point, breast cancer can occur even in those with a long track record of normal imaging. As a general guideline, screening may be stopped when a woman's life expectancy is less than 10 years, but this decision should be highly individualized and based on a thoughtful conversation with your doctor.

And here's something worth emphasizing: not having a family history of breast cancer doesn't mean you're off the hook. While it's true that having a first-degree relative with breast cancer increases your personal risk, most women diagnosed with breast cancer-about 85 to 90%-have no family history at all (Collaborative Group, *The Lancet*, 1997; Durham et al., 2022). They become, in a sense, the start of their family history. So, skipping screening because "no one in my family had it" is not just a flawed assumption; it can be dangerous. Your diagnosis might be the one that protects someone you love by encouraging earlier or more attentive screening for them.

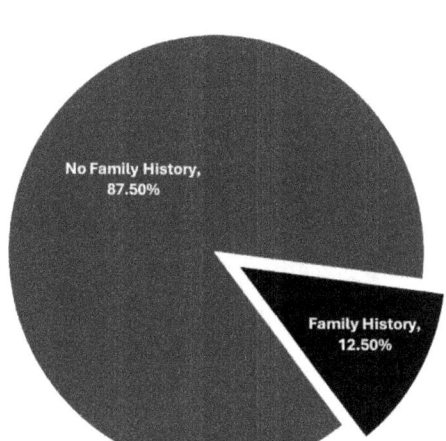

Breast Cancer Diagnosis and Family History of Breast Cancer

No Family History, 87.50%

Family History, 12.50%

Breast cancer screening is not about fear; it's about empowerment. It's about using the tools we have to find trouble early, when we have the most options and the greatest chance of success. Like many forms of health maintenance, it's a small effort that can make a life-changing difference.

Screening for Colon Cancer

Colorectal cancer is both common and detectable, making it one of the most important cancers to screen for. The United States Preventive Services Task Force (USPSTF) recommends that screening begin at age 45 for people at average risk (meaning no personal or family history of colon cancer, no genetic predisposition, and no inflammatory bowel disease like

Crohn's or ulcerative colitis). For those with additional risk factors, including family history or certain inherited conditions, screening may need to begin earlier. In this book, we will focus on what applies to the general population.

There are several ways to screen, and each comes with its own strengths:

- Fecal Immunochemical Test (FIT): This stool-based test checks for hidden blood in the stool and is done once a year.
- Stool DNA test (like Cologuard ©): This combines FIT with DNA markers that may indicate cancer or pre-cancer and is done every three years.
- Colonoscopy: Often considered the gold standard, this is a direct visualization procedure that allows doctors not only to detect but also to remove precancerous growths during the same visit. This is my preferred test to screen for colorectal cancer.

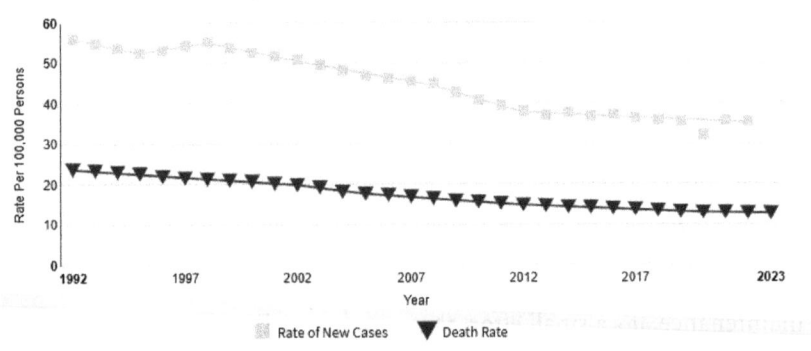

Image: Colorectal cancer new cases (56 per 100,000 in 1992 to 35 per 100,000 in 2023) and death rate (decreased from 23.7 to 12.7 per 100,000 from 1992 to 2023 in the US).

Source: National Cancer Institute (NCI)

Let's take a closer look at colonoscopy. During this procedure, a long, flexible tube with a tiny camera (called a colonoscope) is inserted through the rectum to examine the inside of the colon. Patients take a bowel prep the day before to clean out the colon completely, ensuring the doctor has a clear view. Most people receive light sedation for comfort, and the procedure typically takes between 30 and 60 minutes. The real power of colonoscopy lies in its triple benefit: it can screen, diagnose, and treat all in one procedure.

This is important because most colorectal cancers begin as adenomatous polyps: small, benign growths that slowly transform into cancer over the course of about 10 years. These polyps are found in approximately 30% of men and 20% of women over the age of 40. Catching them early and removing them is how we stop cancer before it ever starts.

The follow-up timeline for your next colonoscopy depends on what's found during the first. If no polyps are found, you may not need another for 10 years. But if polyps are detected, the next exam might be in 3 to 5 years, depending on their number, size, and features under the microscope.

Now, not everyone is comfortable with the idea of a colonoscopy, and that's okay and understandable. The stool-based options are perfectly valid and meaningful alternatives. In my own practice, if I sense reluctance or notice that a previously ordered colonoscopy wasn't completed, I pivot to a stool test. What matters most is that screening happens and that we have a plan in place if a test comes back positive. In that case, a diagnostic colonoscopy becomes the necessary next step.

As for when to stop screening, general guidelines recommend continuing at least through age 75. Beyond that, it becomes a personalized decision based on your overall health, prior test results, and estimated life expectancy of 10 years or more. Again, this is where the value of a primary care team comes into play-they help navigate what's best for you.

A common question I hear is: *"What if I don't have a family history of colon cancer?"* And yes, having a close relative diagnosed at a young age does increase your personal risk. But data from the American Cancer Society (2023) suggests that about 30% of people diagnosed with colorectal cancer do have a family history, which means 70% do not. Just like with breast cancer, many people become the first case in their family. They become, if I may, *their family history.* Skipping screening just because no one else in your family had it is a false sense of reassurance and can delay lifesaving detection. Your diagnosis could be the one that opens the door to early awareness and testing for your children, siblings, or loved ones.

Yes, I've used a similar message here as I did in the breast cancer section, and that's on purpose. In real conversations with patients, this framing makes a difference. It reframes the role of screening not just as an individual decision, but as an act that can ripple outward to protect the people we care about.

Colon cancer is common. But so is the ability to catch it early or stop it entirely. And that's why screening matters.

Screening for Prostate Cancer

Let's begin with a basic question: What is the prostate? The prostate is a small, walnut-sized gland found only in men, sitting just below the bladder and in front of the rectum. Its main role is to produce seminal fluid, which helps nourish and transport sperm. As men age, the prostate often changes; it can become enlarged or, in some cases, develop cancer. Prostate cancer is one of the most common cancers in men and a leading cause of cancer-related death among males in the United States.

It's important to know that prostate size doesn't always tell the full story. An enlarged prostate is very common with aging and is usually due to a non-cancerous condition called benign prostatic hyperplasia (BPH). BPH can cause urinary symptoms and is often the reason men seek medical care. On the other hand, prostate cancer is frequently asymptomatic in its early stages, and many men with prostate cancer have a "normal-sized" prostate. So, the size of the prostate does not reliably predict the presence or absence of cancer.

The primary tool for prostate cancer screening is a blood test called PSA, which stands for "prostate-specific antigen". PSA is an enzyme produced by prostate cells. While rising levels can suggest prostate cancer, they can also increase due to non-cancerous causes, such as inflammation, infection, recent ejaculation, prostate manipulation (like during a rectal exam), or even activities like cycling. Age, medications, and prostate volume can all influence PSA levels. That's why PSA results must be interpreted in context, not just by a lab number, but through an informed conversation with your healthcare provider.

You might have heard about the digital rectal exam (DRE) as part of a "complete exam." While it has historically been part of prostate evaluation, DRE is no longer recommended as a routine screening tool, either on its own or alongside PSA. Why? Because it only accesses the back and side areas of the prostate, not the whole gland, and its accuracy depends heavily on the examiner's technique and experience. It's still useful in certain clinical scenarios, but not as a primary screening method.

One source of confusion for many patients is the overlap in location between prostate cancer and colorectal cancer. Both may involve rectal exams, and both cancers occur in the lower pelvis, but they are entirely different diseases. Colorectal cancer affects the digestive system, while prostate cancer affects the genito-urinary system. They require different screening strategies, apply to different age groups, and serve different purposes. Understanding the difference and ensuring both screenings are done when appropriate can be lifesaving.

Prostate cancer screening is not "one-size-fits-all". Unlike some other cancer screenings that are universally recommended, PSA testing is highly individualized. Most men should begin discussing prostate cancer screening with their doctor around age 50, but those at higher risk, such as Black men or those with a first-degree relative who had prostate cancer before age 65, should start that conversation earlier, sometime around age 45.

And here's where shared decision-making becomes especially important. While early detection can save lives, PSA screening also carries the risk of overdiagnosis-detecting slow-growing cancers that may never cause symptoms or shorten life. Treatment for these cancers can carry side effects, including incontinence and erectile dysfunction. Therefore, rather than offering blanket advice, the best approach is to discuss the pros and cons with your doctor. Together, you can consider your age, values, health status, and family history to decide whether, when, and how to screen.

If the decision is made to pursue screening, PSA is usually monitored every 1–2 years. When trends are stable and there's no cause for concern, longer intervals are often fine. However, if the PSA is elevated or shows a concerning trend, further evaluation may include repeat testing, imaging (such as a prostate MRI), or referral to a specialist (a urologist).

In short, prostate cancer screening is not just a test; it's a conversation. It's about knowing your body, understanding your risks, and working with your healthcare team to make decisions that fit your life. Screening doesn't mean rushing to treatment. It means staying informed, staying engaged, and making room for prevention before problems arise.

Shared Decision-Making for PSA Screening

Prostate cancer screening with the **PSA (prostate-specific antigen)** test isn't universally recommended for all men. Unlike screenings where the benefit clearly outweighs the risk for most people, PSA testing falls into a more nuanced category. That's why the decision to screen should be grounded in a thoughtful, personalized conversation between a patient and their healthcare provider. This isn't a checkbox, it's a dialogue.

Here's a brief overview of the potential benefits and harms to help guide that decision:

Potential Benefits of PSA Screening	Potential Harms of PSA Screening
Early detection of prostate cancer	False positives leading to anxiety and further testing
Treatment when cancer is more curable	Detection of slow-growing cancer that may never cause symptoms
Peace of mind for some individuals	Side effects from biopsy (bleeding, infection)
May reduce the risk of cancer spreading	Side effects from treatment (incontinence, erectile dysfunction, extreme fatigue)

To help frame this in more intuitive terms, let's return to the barnyard metaphor: imagine trying to keep a turtle, rabbit, and bird in a barn. The bird escapes almost instantly, just like an aggressive cancer that grows and spreads before a test can catch it. The rabbit might get away quickly, but with timely screening, it can often be caught. These are the cancers we aim to detect. The turtle, though, moves so slowly that even with the barn door wide open, it may never leave. Many prostate cancers in older adults behave like turtles: slow-growing and unlikely to cause harm in one's lifetime.

This is why most guidelines, including those from the American Urological Association, recommend against routine PSA screening in men over age 70. The potential for overdiagnosis and overtreatment increases, while the chance of the cancer causing serious harm decreases. There's even a saying among doctors: "Many men die with prostate cancer, not of it."

That said, I don't believe in hard cutoffs. In my practice, I prefer to individualize the decision. Age alone doesn't tell the full story. A healthy, active 72-year-old with a long life expectancy may still benefit from continued screening, especially if they value early detection. Conversely, for someone with multiple chronic conditions or limited life expectancy, screening may do more harm than good.

And once again, this is where the role of a primary care provider becomes invaluable. A doctor who knows your story, your health history, preferences, and values is best equipped to guide you through this decision. Continuity of care, year after year, allows for conversations that evolve with time, not just snapshots based on age or lab numbers.

Screening for Lung Cancer

Lung cancer remains one of the leading causes of cancer-related death in both men and women. One of the most powerful tools we have to reduce that burden is screening, particularly for people at high risk due to smoking history.

The U.S. Preventive Services Task Force (USPSTF) recommends annual screening with low-dose computed tomography (LDCT) for adults aged 50 to 80 who meet the following criteria:

- They have at least a **20 pack-year** smoking history (meaning they smoked one pack a day for 20 years, or two packs a day for 10 years).
- And they either **currently smoke** or **have quit within the past 15 years.**

Screening should be discontinued once a person has gone 15 years without smoking or develops health conditions that significantly limit life expectancy or the ability to undergo curative lung surgery. The goal here isn't just to find cancer; it's to find it while it's still small, localized, and treatable.

LDCT is a game-changer in this space. It's far more sensitive than a standard chest X-ray and can detect tiny nodules long before symptoms arise. The National Lung Screening Trial (NLST) showed that LDCT screening reduced lung cancer deaths by 20% compared to chest X-rays.

But the benefits don't stop at the lungs. These scans can incidentally pick up other important health findings, like coronary artery calcifications, which are markers of atherosclerosis. Identifying these can offer an opportunity to assess cardiovascular risk and intervene early, perhaps with lifestyle changes, medications, or further testing. It's a perfect example of how screening, while aimed at one disease, can have a ripple effect to improve health in other areas.

There's also a subtle but profound behavioral benefit. For some patients, the act of undergoing a lung cancer screening, especially when they see images of their lungs or hear a concerning result, can serve as a powerful motivator to quit smoking. It turns a theoretical risk into something concrete and personal. And that moment of clarity can be the beginning of real change.

It's worth noting that chest X-rays, once used for screening, are no longer recommended for this purpose. Research, including the landmark PLCO trial (Oken et al., 2011), has shown that chest X-rays do not significantly reduce mortality from lung cancer. Simply put, they're not sensitive enough to catch disease early, and relying on them may lead to false reassurance.

In summary, LDCT is the gold standard for lung cancer screening in high-risk individuals. It offers the opportunity to catch cancer early, spot other hidden risks, and, perhaps most importantly, start a conversation about quitting smoking and protecting long-term health. Like all screening, it's not a standalone event; it is part of a broader commitment to staying ahead of disease before it ever knocks on the door.

Immunizations

If there's one tool in modern medicine that has transformed public health more than almost any other, it's vaccination. The immunization schedules currently recommended in the United States (as of May 2025) are based on decades of rigorous research and real-world evidence, consistently demonstrating both their effectiveness and safety. While this book is not intended to delve deeply into each specific vaccine or navigate the controversies that have surfaced in recent years, it is worth pausing to reflect on the remarkable impact that vaccines have had on human health and to ground that understanding in data, rather than headlines.

The full, up-to-date immunization schedule is easily accessible at cdc.gov, and is tailored by age, health status, pregnancy, and medical risk factors. Instead of detailing every vaccine here, I want to share several major studies that highlight the global scale of vaccine benefits:

- A 2024 World Health Organization (WHO) report found that global immunization efforts over the past 50 years have saved 154 million lives, with 95% of those lives being children under the age of five. On average, each life saved translates to 66 additional years of health, totaling more than **10.2 billion healthy life** years gained. Polio vaccination alone enabled over 20 million people to walk who would have otherwise been paralyzed. Measles vaccination accounted for an estimated 60% of lives saved, highlighting its profound role in reducing infant and childhood mortality.
- A study published by the Centers for Disease Control and Prevention (Zhou et al., 2024) evaluated the health and economic outcomes of routine childhood vaccinations in the U.S. across 30 birth cohorts (1994–2023). The results were striking: vaccines prevented 508 million illnesses, 32 million hospitalizations, and 1.1 million deaths. Financially, these efforts translated into $540

billion in direct savings and $2.7 trillion in broader societal savings.

- A massive global study (Faksova et al., 2024), **involving 99 million people**, looked at COVID-19 vaccine safety. Across more than 183 million vaccine doses, mild and self-limiting events, such as myocarditis and pericarditis, were observed, particularly in younger men; however, these occurred far less frequently than the same conditions following a COVID-19 infection. A study by Frontera et al. (2022) found that neurological complications after COVID infection were up to **617 times more common** than after COVID vaccination. That's not a rounding error; it is a message: the disease is far more dangerous than the shot.

One of the most exciting examples of vaccines actively preventing cancer comes from the HPV vaccine. Human papillomavirus (HPV) is a known cause of cervical, anal, and head and neck cancers. Widespread HPV vaccination has had such a significant impact that Sweden is now on track to eradicate cervical cancer by 2027, a milestone previously thought impossible (Swedish Cancer Society). Denmark has also announced progress toward eliminating cervical cancer by 2040, thanks to a national effort combining HPV vaccination with strong cervical cancer screening programs (Danish Cancer Society).

Despite all this evidence, conversations about vaccines, especially the COVID-19 vaccine, often include stories. A neighbor who had a heart attack after a shot. A friend of a friend who developed a blood clot or a seizure. These stories are powerful, and I hear them often. The emotional impact of hearing that something bad happened to someone you know can easily outweigh a pile of data. But when we step back and look at the broader picture, the story changes.

Yes, people sometimes experience health events shortly after vaccination. But that doesn't mean the vaccine caused them. **Life continues after a vaccine.** People still have heart attacks, strokes, and accidents. They still get sick for unrelated reasons. The job of public health is to look not just at **what happened**, but whether it happened **more often than expected**. And when we compare the **observed rates** of adverse events post-vaccination to what we'd expect in any large group of people, we almost always find that **the rates are similar**. In other words, these events were likely going to happen anyway.

To bring this home, imagine someone getting hit by a car two days after receiving a flu shot. No one would blame the vaccine. But if they had a heart attack two days later, the connection feels easier to make, even if it's just as coincidental. **Our minds are wired to look for patterns, but science is designed to verify them.**

Vaccines are not perfect. But neither is life. What they offer is protection from diseases that were once feared, deadly, and common, and they do it with an incredible safety record. Millions of lives have been saved, childhood death rates have plummeted, cancer rates are falling in specific populations, and infections that once devastated communities are now preventable.

And that, more than anything else, is why immunizations are a cornerstone of health maintenance, not just for individuals, but for society as a whole.

Sleep

One expert once called the sleep-loss epidemic "the greatest public health challenge of the twenty-first century." That may sound dramatic, but the data backs it up. In a world that rewards productivity, busyness, and round-the-clock connectivity, sleep is often the first thing we sacrifice. Yet it's one of the most important pillars of health, on par with diet and exercise, and just as easy to ignore.

According to a consensus statement by the American Academy of Sleep Medicine and the Sleep Research Society, adults aged 18 to 60 should aim for at least **seven hours of sleep** per night. This isn't about luxury or laziness, it's about function, repair, and long-term wellbeing. Regularly falling short of that threshold can affect more than just your mood. Symptoms of sleep deprivation include irritability, daytime fatigue, impaired memory and concentration, and, of course, overwhelming sleepiness. But the effects run deeper than that.

Sleep is essential for both brain function and physical health. While we rest, our bodies regulate hormones, repair tissues, balance our immune system, and, most fascinatingly, clear waste from the brain, a process that only occurs efficiently during deep sleep. This is the brain's night shift: clearing out neurotoxic debris like beta-amyloid, the same substance associated with Alzheimer's disease. Getting enough sleep, especially deep, high-quality sleep, isn't just about feeling refreshed the next day. It's about protecting your heart, memory, metabolism, and emotional resilience.

We cycle through three key stages of sleep:

- Light sleep, where the body begins to wind down, is characterized by a drop in temperature and heart rate.
- Deep sleep, the most restorative phase, essential for muscle repair, immune regulation, and brain detoxification.
- REM sleep, where most dreaming occurs, plays a key role in mood regulation and memory consolidation.

All three are necessary, but deep sleep is particularly valuable for overall health.

Today, many people are using wearable devices, like the Oura© ring, Apple© Watch, Fitbit©, and others, to track their sleep. While not perfectly accurate, these tools are powerful awareness builders. They help users detect trends, explore correlations (like how meal timing or alcohol affects sleep), and open doors to conversations with physicians. Some even have the ability to detect signs of **possible sleep apnea**, a common but often underdiagnosed condition.

Sleep Apnea – A Closer Look

Sleep apnea is a condition where breathing stops and restarts repeatedly during sleep, resulting in fragmented, poor-quality rest and drops in oxygen levels overnight (NIH).

- Snoring is a common symptom, but not all snorers have sleep apnea, and some people with apnea don't snore at all.
- It's often associated with excess weight, but can also occur in individuals with normal body mass. Conversely, some overweight individuals never develop it.
- Warning signs include daytime sleepiness, fatigue, morning headaches, uncontrolled high blood pressure, and detection of abnormal sleep patterns by wearables.
- Left untreated, sleep apnea increases the risk for heart disease, atrial fibrillation, pulmonary hypertension, and accidents related to daytime fatigue, such as falling asleep while driving or operating machinery.

Diagnosis is typically made through a home sleep study or a formal sleep lab test, and treatment options range from CPAP machines to oral devices or weight management strategies.

In clinical practice, I've seen how small changes can yield big benefits. Simply setting a consistent bedtime, even 30 minutes earlier, can make a significant difference in how people feel and perform. And while many think they need eight hours, research suggests that for most adults, seven is the sweet spot, especially when that time includes plenty of deep sleep.

According to the CDC, here are some key habits to support better sleep:

- Go to bed and wake up at the same time every day, even on weekends.
- Keep your bedroom quiet, dark, cool, and relaxing.
- Avoid screens (TV, phone, tablet) for at least 30 minutes before bedtime.
- Skip large meals, alcohol, and caffeine in the late afternoon or evening.
- Stay physically active and follow a healthy diet.

If you're struggling with sleep, a great first step is keeping a sleep diary. Track when you go to bed and wake up, how many times you wake at night, your caffeine and alcohol intake, your screen time, and what you ate and when. Bring this diary to your primary care provider; you may discover a pattern or open the door to further evaluation and solutions.

Sleep isn't wasted time. It's protective, productive, and necessary. Treat it like a health priority.

Primary Care Physician Role

With the risk of sounding biased, as a primary care physician myself, I truly believe that having a primary care doctor is one of the simplest investments a patient can make in their long-term health. Think of the PCP as the quarterback of the medical team: someone who knows the playbook, keeps track of the whole field, and helps patients make smart moves to stay healthy. In this section, we'll talk about what to expect from a primary care relationship, why it matters, and how the system is evolving.

Unfortunately, we're facing a national shortage of primary care doctors in the U.S., and the future doesn't look much brighter. The Association of American Medical Colleges (AAMC) estimates we will experience a **shortage of 20,000 to 40,000 primary care physicians** by 2036. Increasingly, care is delivered by a team: a physician working alongside advanced practice providers like nurse practitioners (NPs) and physician assistants (PAs) and a nursing team. This team allows more patients to receive longitudinal care and is a perfect option when done by the right people in the right setting.

That said, not every sore throat or sprained ankle needs to go through your primary doctor. There are plenty of options for quick, convenient visits—walk-in clinics, urgent care centers, and telehealth services—for those simpler, one-off concerns, such as a cold, flu, or urinary infection. However, when something is recurring, unexplained, or part of a chronic condition, such as persistent fever, ongoing cough, abdominal pain, abnormal lab results, weight loss, or managing blood pressure or diabetes, among others, that's when the PCP and their team should be the first point of contact. They're the ones who see the full picture.

Communication is everything. Many healthcare systems now utilize secure online portals that allow patients to send messages, view test results, and stay connected between visits. This adds to the continuity and fluency of the patient-primary care-physician connection.

One of the greatest threats to long-term, trusting relationships in primary care isn't medical, it's financial. Insurance coverage, or more precisely, the way it shifts year to year, can disrupt even the most well-established doctor-patient partnerships. Each open enrollment season brings a wave of changes: employer plan switches, marketplace reshuffling, cost hikes, network alterations. And suddenly, patients who've built years of care with a trusted physician find themselves out of network or are forced to start over elsewhere.

I see this all the time, and it never gets easier. I'm humbled by the patients who go out of their way to adjust their insurance just to stay within our network. That choice isn't small; it often comes with a higher premium or limited options elsewhere. And I also fully understand and never judge those who can't. Sometimes, the incentives and financial pressures are too heavy to ignore, especially for families or those navigating job changes. Healthcare is expensive, and no one should be made to feel guilty for choosing what they can afford.

Still, this reality underscores another reason why continuity tools like patient portals are so important. Even when formal coverage changes, patients often stay in touch, sharing updates, asking for input, or even just letting me know how they're doing. These digital threads help maintain a connection, a sense of consistency. And on those rare but joyful days when someone writes to say they've switched plans again and can come back under my care, it's like seeing an old friend walk through the door.

Primary care works best as a longitudinal partnership, a relationship built over time, year after year. It's not just about checkboxes or prescriptions. Over time, the conversations deepen, the trust grows, and we build a kind of professional friendship rooted in shared goals: keeping you well-informed, and in control.

Now, let's talk about the patient's role. Every patient should feel empowered to ask for their records. By law, medical practices must provide them upon request. A single patient can generate up to **80 to 100 megabytes of data each year** (labs, imaging, notes), especially with modern CT and MRI technology. Over a lifetime, that's several gigabytes of information that may be scattered across systems. And because most medical institutions are only required to retain these records for **seven years** after the last visit (and that varies by state), it's wise to keep your own archive.

Here's a simple checklist of what to bring to an appointment with a new doctor:

- Lab test results from the past 2–3 years.
- Most recent colonoscopy and its pathology report.
- Most recent mammogram.
- Immunization records.
- Imaging test reports from the past 3 years.
- Home blood pressure values - if taking blood pressure medications.
- Any report for a test that your prior doctor(s) said needs repeating.

Ideally, have both the report and the image disc for imaging tests. That way, if you move, switch clinicians, or see a new specialist, your care doesn't start from scratch; it builds on a solid foundation.

Your PCP isn't just your doctor; they're your anchor in the system. And in a fragmented, fast-moving world of healthcare, having someone who knows you, and who walks with you year after year, can make all the difference.

Social Connection and Its Health Power

Health isn't just about what you eat, how often you exercise, or what medications you take; it's also deeply shaped by your social life. Humans are wired for connection, and staying socially engaged brings powerful benefits to both body and mind. People who regularly spend time with family, friends, or a community group tend to have lower rates of depression, better immune responses, and even improved memory. Socializing stimulates the brain, keeps neural circuits engaged, and helps reduce stress and inflammation, which are both linked to chronic disease and cognitive decline.

One of the clearest examples of this can be found in the Blue Zones, regions around the world where people consistently live into their 90s and beyond with good health. Places like Okinawa, Japan and Sardinia, Italy don't just feature healthy diets and daily activity; they also place tremendous value on social connection. Elders in these regions stay deeply integrated into community life, supported by strong social networks that offer purpose and belonging. Researchers have found that this sense of connection may be just as critical to longevity as nutrition or exercise.

Social connection can also take the form of spiritual or religious engagement. A well-known study published in *JAMA Internal Medicine* (Li et al., 2016) included 74,534 women (data collected as part of the Nurses' Health Study), found that those who attended religious services regularly had a 33% lower all-cause mortality, a 27% lower cardiovascular mortality, and a 21% lower cancer mortality. While the benefit likely comes from multiple sources, such as shared values, emotional support, and a sense of purpose, it reminds us that community, in any form, is medicine. Whether it's a walking group, a book club, or weekly worship, meaningful social interaction isn't a luxury; it's a tool for a longer, healthier life.

They reflect the consensus in the literature about how social connection contributes to different domains of health, but they are not exact measurements or effect sizes. Here are other aspects that reflect the role of social connections:

1. **Cognitive Health**

    Social engagement is consistently linked to better memory and reduced dementia risk. For example, a study measured the level of amyloid-beta (marker of Alzheimer's disease) and noted an association between social engagement and the rate of decline in amyloid-beta (Biddle et al, 2019). Krueger et al (2009) confirm that higher levels of social integration are associated with better cognition.

2. **Emotional Wellbeing**

    Strong social connections are significant protective factors against depression and anxiety. A comprehensive review study by Wickramaratne et al. (2022) demonstrates that social support ameliorates symptoms of depression. Conversely, feelings of loneliness are associated with an increased risk of major depressive disorder.

3. **Physical Health**

    Social isolation is associated with increased inflammation (Matthews et al., 2024). We are starting to advance again in the M3 complex of diseases territory, with data from another study (Parker et al, 2024) indicating that social isolation in young/early adulthood increased the odds of hypertension.

4. **Longevity**

    This rating is supported by both observations from Blue Zones and large cohort studies. A meta-analysis published in PLOS Medicine (Holt-Lunstad et al., 2010) showed that strong social relationships increase the likelihood of survival by 50%. The authors describe the impact of social connections as comparable to that of well-known risk factors such as alcohol and tobacco use.

In the end, social connection isn't just a feel-good bonus; it's a central pillar of good health. The evidence is clear: meaningful relationships protect our minds, sharpen our memories, and strengthen our hearts. People who stay socially engaged experience lower rates of depression and anxiety, better cognitive performance as they age, and even reduced risks of high blood pressure, heart disease, and stroke. From conversations over coffee to participating in religious services or community groups, these interactions buffer stress, lower inflammation, and offer a deep sense of purpose. In a world where isolation has quietly become a health threat, choosing connection may be one of the most powerful and most human forms of prevention we have.

Summary

Health maintenance is where everything comes together. It's not about chasing perfection, but about building consistency —small actions taken over time that quietly protect us before we ever feel unwell. Through screenings, immunizations, sleep, social connection, and a relationship with a primary care team, we create a health strategy rooted in prevention, awareness, and self-respect. We've seen that most chronic conditions don't arrive overnight; they take shape slowly, quietly, often in the background. That's why this chapter has focused on what we can do in that quiet space before symptoms appear. Whether it's detecting cancer early, preventing infectious disease, managing stress and sleep, or staying connected to people who make life meaningful, the best medicine is often the one that keeps us from needing medicine at all. Health maintenance isn't a task list; it's a mindset. And in the long arc of a life, it may be one of the most powerful tools we have to shape our outcome.

CHAPTER 9

Exploring Additional Health Claims

We've covered the fundamentals: diet, movement, medication, and the major players in disease prevention. But what about everything else? The wellness world is filled with products and practices that promise better health, ranging from supplements and genetic tests to full-body scans and detox regimens. Some of these ideas come up regularly in conversation, in clinics, and on social media, often with more marketing than medicine behind them. This chapter is meant to walk through those "other ideas," not with judgment, but with clarity. What's worth considering? What's just noise? And how do we stay open-minded without getting misled? Let's take a closer look.

No Magic Pill

Let's start with the uncomfortable truth: there is no magic solution. No shortcut to undoing years of metabolic strain or reversing the risks tied to the M3 cluster-metabolic disease, malignancy, and memory impairment. No drink, pill, or trendy program is going to single-handedly solve it.

You've probably seen the commercials: smiling people, often celebrities, holding colorful bottles of "natural" energy boosters, memory enhancers, and metabolism boosters. The packaging is usually green, the word "natural" is repeated like a mantra, and the results sound miraculous.

Let's pause there. "Natural?" It's a word that's been stretched beyond recognition. Something produced in a factory, sealed in a plastic bottle, pressed into a pill, and shipped in bulk-that's not natural. That's industrial. Real natural is a blueberry. A walnut. A head of broccoli. Something you can grow, pick, and eat without needing a disclaimer.

And speaking of disclaimers, flip the bottle over and look closely. There's often a tiny asterisk followed by a sentence like: *"This product has not been evaluated by the FDA and is not intended to diagnose, treat, cure, or prevent any disease."* That little line is doing a lot of heavy lifting. It basically tells you: we don't know if this works, and no one has tested it the way prescription medicines are tested.

So, what does it take for something to be evaluated and approved by the FDA (Food and Drug Administration)? A lot. Years of research, clinical trials involving thousands of people, rigorous safety reviews, and detailed analysis of how the drug interacts with other medications. That's why FDA-approved medications come with long pamphlets and even longer TV ads listing potential side effects. Ironically, that very transparency, meant to protect you, often scares people off. Meanwhile, the untested "natural" product with zero safety data gets a free pass.

To be clear, most over-the-counter supplements are likely harmless, though many are also likely ineffective or minimally beneficial. But some *can* cause harm, especially when mixed with other medications, or taken in high doses, or assumed to be a fix-all.

Here's the bottom line: there's no magic pill for weight loss, or cholesterol control, or better energy. Real progress takes effort. It takes time. And it almost always happens at the individual level, with guidance from professionals, yes, but built on your own decisions. The good news? It *is* possible. And the return on that investment is not just better numbers on a lab test; it's a better life, better function, and more time to enjoy it.

Supplements

Let's be honest: supplements come up a *lot*. In casual conversations, in media headlines, and in my clinic. Many patients walk in already taking a handful of capsules they've picked up based on advice from friends, influencers, or the local health food store. Others ask whether they *should* be taking something "just in case." So, let's slow down and walk through a few of the most discussed supplements, ones that come up regularly in my practice.

This isn't an exhaustive list, and I'm not here to dismiss supplements altogether. Some of them *do* have a role. But it's important to put them into perspective: What do they do? What don't they do? And when are they helpful?

Red Yeast Rice

Red yeast rice is often described as a "natural" cholesterol-lowering supplement, but what's not widely advertised is that it contains monacolin K, the very same compound found in the prescription drug **lovastatin**. They are identical from a chemical standpoint. In essence, red yeast rice *is* a statin. Just a weaker, unregulated version.

That matters. Because statins, while incredibly effective and well-studied, do have potential side effects, and red yeast rice is no exception. People can still experience muscle aches, liver enzyme elevations, or interactions with other medications. But unlike prescription statins, red yeast rice isn't standardized. The amount of active compound varies wildly from bottle to bottle. That means inconsistent results and unclear safety.

If you're going to use a statin, you might as well use one that's been rigorously tested, FDA-approved, and dosed precisely. Prescription statins can be tailored to your needs, monitored with lab work, and adjusted safely. Red yeast rice skips all of that. For most patients, it's not the safer or smarter route; it's just the *less regulated* one.

Coenzyme Q10 (CoQ10)

CoQ10 is a naturally occurring antioxidant that plays a key role in energy production within our cells. It's become popular as a supplement, particularly among people taking statins. The theory is that since statins may lower CoQ10 levels in the body, supplementing might prevent or ease muscle aches.

Unfortunately, while it sounds good in theory, the evidence hasn't panned out. A meta-analysis on 6 randomized control trials (Banach et al., 2015) concluded that coenzyme Q10 did not provide a significant benefit in statin-related muscle symptoms. If there is any benefit, it's likely minimal or placebo.

That doesn't mean it's harmful, but it may not be worth the cost or the pill burden if you're hoping it will "fix" statin side effects. As always, talk to your doctor before trying it.

Turmeric

Turmeric is a golden-yellow spice, most often found in curry dishes, but also in supplement aisles, usually in the form of curcumin, its active compound. It's been studied for its anti-inflammatory properties and may offer modest relief for conditions like osteoarthritis or general musculoskeletal pain.

While it's not a replacement for other therapies, some people do report benefits from taking turmeric or curcumin supplements. If it works for you and causes no harm, that's fine. Please note that high doses may interact with blood thinners, and not all supplements are created equal in terms of purity and absorption.

Vitamin B Complex

Vitamin B12

Vitamin B12 is essential for nerve function and red blood cell production. Deficiencies are more common than people think, especially among vegans, individuals with malabsorption conditions (like celiac or pernicious anemia), or those taking metformin for type 2 diabetes.

One indicator of B12 deficiency in labs may be macrocytosis, a finding on lab tests where red blood cells appear larger than normal. B12 deficiency can also present with neuropathy, manifested through numbness, tingling, or balance issues.

Supplementing with B12 is generally safe and effective. In fact, it's hard to overdose, but very high levels may not provide extra benefit, and occasionally they can mask other problems. It's reasonable to check levels in at-risk individuals or those with suggestive symptoms.

Vitamin B6

Vitamin B6 helps with brain development and immune function. Deficiency, though uncommon, can result from alcohol use disorder, certain medications, or kidney disease. Symptoms may include irritability, depression, or nerve-related issues.

Supplementation is helpful when needed, but excess B6 over long periods can *also* cause nerve damage. So more isn't always better.

Vitamin B1 (Thiamine)

Thiamine deficiency is rarer but can be serious, especially in alcohol use disorder or in people with chronic malnutrition or severe vomiting. It's classically linked to Wernicke's encephalopathy, a neurologic emergency that affects balance, eye movements, and memory.

Thiamine supplements are safe and often given proactively in hospitals when risk factors are present.

Vitamin D

Vitamin D is important for bone health, calcium absorption, and immune function. We get it from sun exposure, certain foods (like fatty fish or fortified milk), and supplements.

Deficiency can occur in people with limited sun exposure, darker skin tones, or malabsorption syndromes. For the most part, vitamin D deficiency is asymptomatic unless it persists over a prolonged period.

However, there's a growing recognition that routine screening for vitamin D in healthy, asymptomatic adults offers no clear benefit. Major guidelines suggest not testing unless there's a clinical reason.

Once supplementation begins, it's reasonable to monitor levels occasionally to ensure effectiveness and avoid excess. But in general, blindly checking vitamin D "just to see" hasn't been shown to improve outcomes, and it can add to healthcare costs without adding value.

Final Thoughts about Supplements

Supplements aren't inherently bad and, in some cases, they're necessary. But they should be used with care, not casually. "Natural" does not always mean better, and "more" does not always mean safer. Always ask: *Why am I taking this? Do I need it? Is there something better studied or more effective?*

Supplements can *support* a healthy lifestyle, but they can't replace the basics: a balanced diet, regular movement, adequate sleep, and personalized medical care. In the end, health isn't built on bottles or pills, it's built on habits.

CT or MRI Scan of the Whole Body

This idea comes up more and more, often from a well-meaning place. A patient wants to be proactive, catch things early, and feel in control. They've heard of someone who got a full-body scan, "just to be safe," and wonder: *Should I do the same?*

It's an understandable instinct. But here's the reality: **whole-body CT or MRI scans are not recommended by clinical guidelines** for healthy, asymptomatic individuals.

Why not? Let's bring back the metaphor I used previously: the barnyard and the bird. Once a bird has flown out of the barn, shutting the doors won't help catch it. Similarly, a full-body scan may give the illusion that everything is fine, but it won't stop something from developing after the scan. It's a moment in time, not a guarantee of ongoing health.

That illusion of reassurance can be dangerous. I've seen patients ignore new symptoms—chest pain, fatigue, changes in bowel habits—because "I just had a body scan." But when we dig deeper, the scan was two or three years ago. In medical terms, that's not recent. Diseases don't wait. A scan done in 2022 won't protect you in 2025.

More importantly, the literature does not support the use of full-body imaging in individuals without symptoms or those without specific, high-risk genetic conditions. These tests can miss things they're not optimized to find. For example, a whole-body scan may not detect an early-stage breast tumor that a mammogram would catch. It may overlook a colon polyp or mass that a colonoscopy would reveal. We already have well-established, effective screening tools, tailored to the most common and detectable conditions.

So why are whole-body scans still so popular? Part of it is marketing. These tests are often cash-based and targeted at people who "just want to know."

However, what you're really getting is a snapshot, not a guarantee of health.

And snapshots come with strings attached. One of the biggest concerns with full-body imaging is the discovery of **incidental findings, such as tiny nodules, cysts, or spots,** that almost always turn out to be harmless. But once they're found, they can't be ignored. That sets off a chain of follow-up scans, biopsies, or even surgery, each with its own risks. What begins as curiosity can turn into years of anxiety and procedures. The emotional toll can be heavy, especially when the initial test was never medically necessary.

Whole-body scans are valuable in specific cases, such as staging or monitoring known cancers, or investigating serious unexplained symptoms like unintentional weight loss. In these situations, imaging provides crucial diagnostic information.

However, using these scans routinely in otherwise healthy people adds more cost than value. It's part of a broader issue in U.S. healthcare: we spend more than any other country, but our outcomes don't match the investment. The overuse of advanced imaging contributes to this paradox. It drives up healthcare costs, increases exposure to radiation or unnecessary procedures, and diverts imaging resources away from patients who truly need them, raising prices and lengthening wait times.

When it comes to whole-body scans, the intention is often good, but the execution can backfire. Instead of reassurance, they can bring uncertainty. Instead of prevention, they can bring distraction. In medicine, more testing isn't always better, but smarter testing is. Let's focus on proven screening tools, tailored to individual risk factors, and avoid the trap of testing for the sake of testing.

Peace of mind doesn't come from a scan. It comes from habits, follow-up, trust in your healthcare team and understanding what's worth chasing and what isn't.

Blood Tests for Screening

We live in an age where a simple blood draw can unlock extraordinary amounts of information. It's no wonder that blood-based screening tests, especially those promising early cancer detection, are generating so much buzz. Two types have been making headlines: polygenic risk scores and multi-cancer early detection (MCED) tests. Let's take a closer look at what they are, what they can and can't do, and what science says so far.

Polygenic Risk Scores (PRS)

A polygenic risk score is a type of blood test that analyzes many tiny variations across your DNA, called single-nucleotide polymorphisms (SNPs), to estimate your inherited genetic predisposition to certain diseases. These include common conditions like diabetes, Alzheimer's disease, coronary artery disease, some neurological disorders, and various types of cancer.

Rather than providing a definitive "yes" or "no", the test compares your genetic profile to that of the general population and estimates whether your risk is higher, lower, or about the same. It's a risk *estimation*, not a diagnosis.

These tests have become increasingly accessible, sometimes available for as little as $100 to $200, even from online platforms like Amazon©. But accessibility doesn't equal actionability. While these tests are based on real science, their clinical utility is still being debated. Knowing you have a higher genetic risk doesn't always translate into specific next steps, especially if your lifestyle and lab values are well-managed.

That said, polygenic risk scores may evolve into valuable tools for personalized prevention, especially when combined with traditional risk factors like age, family history, and lab results. But for now, they should be viewed as informational, not prescriptive.

More studies are needed before strong recommendations for or against their widespread use can be made. Interpretation should always be done with care, ideally in consultation with a clinician or genetic counselor who can help put the results into context.

Multi-Cancer Early Detection (MCED) Tests

These tests aim to do something even more ambitious: detect multiple types of cancer with a single blood draw, even before symptoms appear. The science behind them is fascinating. Many cancers release fragments of DNA into the bloodstream, so-called "circulating tumor DNA" (ctDNA). MCED tests are designed to identify this DNA, and in some cases, even predict its tissue of origin.

Sounds groundbreaking, right? And it may well be. But there are a few caveats.

First, these tests are not currently endorsed by major medical guidelines for routine cancer screening. While exciting, they are still largely experimental, and the real-world performance-sensitivity, specificity, false positive values, etc., is still being studied.

Second, while clinical trials are ongoing, there are already case reports suggesting that these tests have helped catch cancer early. A 2024 study by Vittone et al. documented individual cases where asymptomatic patients were diagnosed with early-stage cancers following a positive MCED result. Even more promising, a 2025 study published in *The British Medical Journal* (Rous et al.) concluded that adding MCED tests to standard screening practices could improve early detection rates and patient outcomes.

So, back to our barnyard metaphor, this might be a tool that actually catches the birds before they fly away. That's the hope. But we're not there yet.

It's also worth noting that these tests are generally cash-pay and not inexpensive. As of now, they're marketed directly to consumers and may cost $800 to $1000 or more. That makes access unequal and interpretation inconsistent. A positive test could prompt more invasive testing or procedures, so false positives, overdiagnosis, and patient anxiety remain real concerns.

Final Thoughts

The future of blood-based screening is exciting. We are moving toward a world where your **blood might tell a deeper story,** not just about what's happening now, but what might happen next.

But we're not quite there yet.

These tools (polygenic risk scores and MCED tests) hold promise, but they're still evolving. For now, the best approach is to stay informed, use these tests selectively (and only when they come with expert guidance), and focus on the screening strategies that are already proven: colonoscopies, mammograms, Pap smears, prostate cancer screening discussions, skin checks, and low-dose CT scans for smokers.

In medicine, it's easy to get caught up in the shiny and new. But value doesn't come from novelty; it comes from results. We owe it to ourselves to ask: *Is this test helping me make a better decision, or just giving me more to worry about?*

Cleansing, Detox, and IV Vitamins

There's something inherently appealing about the idea of a reset. The promise of starting fresh, clearing out the bad, and boosting vitality feels intuitive, and it's no surprise that "cleansing" and "detox" programs have exploded in popularity. Juices, teas, powders, pills, and IV drips all claim to flush out toxins, restore balance, and supercharge your health.

But here's the truth: your body already has a detox system, and it works brilliantly.

Your liver, kidneys, gastrointestinal system, skin, and even your lungs are constantly filtering, processing, and removing waste products and potential toxins. That's their job. Unless something is pathologically wrong, there is no scientific basis to suggest that these processes need help from commercial "detox" products.

And the medical literature is clear on this. A comprehensive review (Acosta et al., 2010) found no evidence of health benefits from commercially promoted detox diets or regimens. In fact, there are numerous reports of harm, ranging from electrolyte imbalances and dehydration to liver damage and hospitalization.

Detox Diets and Cleanses

Many detox diets drastically restrict calories, promote rapid weight loss, or rely on unproven herbal formulations. While they may give a short-lived sense of energy or clarity (often just from fasting or a placebo), these regimens are not sustainable, not necessary, and often unsafe.

And, perhaps most importantly, they distract from what really works. Long-term health doesn't come from three days of juice or from a tea that claims to melt belly fat. It comes from consistent habits: real food, movement, sleep, and mental balance.

IV Vitamins: The High-Tech Detox Trend

In recent years, IV vitamin therapy has emerged as the modern upgrade to detox culture. Drip bars, wellness spas, and concierge services offer intravenous infusions that promise to cure hangovers, boost immunity, increase energy, slow aging, and even improve athletic performance.

It sounds high-tech. It looks clinical. But once again, the evidence doesn't live up to the marketing.

IV vitamin drips deliver a mix of water-soluble vitamins (like vitamin C, B-complex, magnesium, sometimes glutathione) directly into the bloodstream. That bypasses the digestive tract, so the idea is you get more immediate absorption. But for most healthy people with no nutritional deficiencies, that extra absorption provides no added benefit.

And there are real risks. IV access always carries the potential for infection, vein irritation (phlebitis), electrolyte imbalances, and, in rare cases, severe allergic reactions or kidney complications. There have been reports of hospitalizations due to improperly mixed infusions, contamination, or dosing errors. These services are often unregulated, especially when offered outside medical settings.

Despite their cost (often $150 to $500 per session), these infusions are almost entirely cash-based. They're rarely covered by insurance because they lack evidence of clinical efficacy. Like many "wellness" products, they're marketed with slick language but little substance, and when things go wrong, the same businesses offering them are rarely equipped to manage the consequences.

Whether it's a detox tea or an IV vitamin drip, the core message remains the same: If it sounds too good to be true, it's probably not true.

There's a billion-dollar industry behind these products, capitalizing on our desire to feel better, live longer, and regain control. But what they offer is the illusion of health, not the real thing.

True detox happens every day, silently and efficiently, in your liver and kidneys. Real energy comes from movement, food, sleep, and connection. And real prevention? It's a long game, built on informed choices, not flashy quick fixes.

Be curious. Ask questions. But know that you don't need to be cleansed, you need to be supported.

Closing Thoughts: Other Ideas

This chapter was never meant to dismiss curiosity; it's meant to guide it. In a world overflowing with health promises, miracle cures, and "just one pill" solutions, it's more important than ever to pause, ask questions, and return to what matters: evidence, experience, and self-awareness.

Whether it's supplements, genetic tests, full-body scans, or vitamin drips, these ideas often start from a good place: a desire to feel better, catch disease early, or stay one step ahead. But good intentions aren't enough. Without solid science behind them, even the most attractive options can end up wasting time, money, or worse, providing false reassurance, delaying care, or adding stress and confusion.

That's why it helps to remember that health isn't something you buy, it's something you build, not with gimmicks or glowing ads, but with real food, movement, sleep, supportive care, and informed decisions. Some tools may help along the way, but only when they're part of a broader, evidence-based strategy.

So stay curious. Keep asking. Keep learning. But also remember: the path to real health rarely comes in a bottle, a drip, or a scan. It comes from the inside out, and it's more sustainable and more empowering than any quick fix could ever offer.

CHAPTER 10

Do It Yourself: How to Set Your Weight Goal and the Diet Plan to Achieve It

If access to a nutritionist was simple and affordable, that would often be the ideal route, offering expert, personalized, and data-driven guidance tailored to each individual's body and lifestyle. But the reality is, nutrition consultations are often not covered by insurance unless a person already has a diagnosis like diabetes. For those trying to prevent illness or reverse early warning signs like prediabetes or weight gain, resources can be frustratingly limited. It reflects a broader, troubling trend: our healthcare system remains treatment-focused rather than prevention-oriented. As a result, many people feel unsupported, give up, and continue down the dangerous path toward the complications of metabolic syndrome.

But we're living in a new era. Thanks to the rise of large language models and artificial intelligence (AI)-powered health tools, we now have the ability to build our own strategies, even without full access to traditional healthcare. These technologies aren't perfect, and I don't claim to be an AI expert, but we'd be missing out if we didn't start making the most of the tools already at our fingertips. So here's how to get started:

Step 1: Get a Digital Scale and Understand Your Body

Start by buying a digital scale; many now sync with your phone to track progress over time. Daily weigh-ins are not about obsession; they're about awareness. When you see a downward trend, it reinforces motivation.

When the trend is upward, it's an early warning that allows for a course correction before a few pounds become ten pounds or more. Everyone responds to foods differently. Your body might gain three pounds overnight from a slice of pizza, while someone else stays the same. Learn your own responses. Identify foods that trigger weight gain and discover those that don't; this becomes your personal weight map.

Weigh yourself daily, ideally in the morning after using the bathroom and before getting dressed. Log it in an app or journal. At the same time, measure your height and calculate your Body Mass Index (BMI). These are your baseline numbers.

Step 2: Set a Realistic Weight Loss Goal

Aim for steady, sustainable progress: no more than 1–2 pounds per week. For example, losing 30 pounds in six months would require an average loss of about 1.1 pounds per week. Let's round it to 1 pound per week for easier math. Sustainability is key; the goal is long-term success, not crash dieting.

Step 3: Calculate Your Total Daily Energy Expenditure (TDEE)

TDEE is the number of calories your body uses per day, factoring in age, weight, height, gender, and physical activity. Use this AI prompt to calculate your TDEE:

"I am ___ years old, ___ gender, weight ___ lbs (or kg), height ___ in (or cm). I exercise ___ times per week. My exercise routine is ___. My job is ___ and involves ___. Calculate my TDEE."

Example Prompt:

"I am a 52-year-old man, 216 lbs, 6'6". I run 3 to 5 miles at a time, 3 times per week and work a sedentary desk job. Calculate my TDEE."

Example Output:

TDEE ≈ 3,061 kcal/day

Step 4: Set Your Caloric Deficit

To lose 1 pound per week, you'll need a deficit of roughly 500 kcal/day from your TDEE.

Example:

TDEE (3,061 kcal) - 500 kcal = 2,561 kcal/day meal plan target

Your daily food intake should stay close to that number. Adjust as needed over time.

Step 5: Design Your Meal Plan

Find a diet that better suits your preferences (see the diet chapter). Use the percentages of macronutrients from that diet (e.g., 30% protein, 40% carbs, 30% fat). You can use an AI assistant to create detailed daily menus based on your preferences.

Sample AI Prompt:

Create a 2,500 kcal/day meal plan with 30% protein, 40% carbs, 30% fat. Include 3 meals and 2 snacks.

Sample Day (Approx. 2,560 kcal):

- **Breakfast (600 kcal):** 3 scrambled eggs, 1 slice whole grain toast, ½ avocado, 1 banana, coffee/tea
- **Snack (300 kcal):** Plain nonfat Greek yogurt, 1 tbsp peanut butter, ½ cup berries
- **Lunch (700 kcal):** Grilled chicken, 1 cup quinoa, roasted vegetables with olive oil, side salad

- **Snack (250 kcal):** Protein shake + 1 apple
- **Dinner (710 kcal):** Baked salmon, ¾ cup brown rice, steamed broccoli, olive oil drizzle, dark chocolate square

You can further customize by prompting:

- "Create a weekly plan with different dinners each night."
- "Exclude almonds and cauliflower."
- "Make a grocery list for this week's plan."
- "Suggest recipes using chicken, quinoa, spinach, and eggs."
- "Use whole foods only."

Step 6: Track Intake Honestly

Life happens-travel, late dinners, work events. Use apps like MacroFactor or MyFitnessPal to stay honest. They teach you what real calories count look like and help you stay within your targets, even if you slip occasionally.

Step 7: Maintain (and Improve) Your Exercise Program

Stick to the exercise routine you used to estimate your TDEE. But don't stop there. Add resistance training to preserve muscle as you lose fat.

Prompts to Use:

- "Create a 3-day/week strength training plan to complement running 3x/week."
- "Give me a weekly workout split for a beginner aiming for fat loss."

Muscle mass is your friend during weight loss-it keeps metabolism at a higher level and supports long-term results.

🎯 Bonus: Stay on Track with AI-Driven Tools

Goal	AI Tool
Log food	MacroFactor, MyFitnessPal
Generate meal plans	ChatGPT, EatThisMuch
Track activity	Apple Watch, Fitbit
Coaching/adjustments	Carbon Diet Coach, MacroFactor
Build habits	Noom, Wysa

Most have free versions. Or use ChatGPT (or other favorite AI assistant); you will have to just type a bit more than using apps.

Final Thoughts

You don't need perfection, you need progress. This DIY approach isn't about being your own doctor or dietitian but about taking agency over your health. The truth is, most of us know what's healthy and what's not. The hard part is structure, accountability, and consistency. Thanks to new tools, we can now build those things ourselves. Prevention isn't passive; it's a choice. And you've just taken the first step toward reclaiming your health on your own terms.

EPILOGUE

The Common Thread, The Common Fix

This book has explored the major chronic diseases that affect our modern lives, including heart attacks and strokes, cancer, and dementia, and laid out a simple yet powerful framework that connects them: **Metabolism, Malignancy, Memory** (M3). These are not isolated conditions; they don't emerge from nowhere. They often grow from the same root.

The evidence is increasingly clear: the same upstream dysfunction-insulin resistance, chronic inflammation, oxidative stress, and poor metabolic health-drives the bulk of chronic disease risk. You don't need three separate strategies to protect your brain, your heart, and your cells. You need to understand the shared drivers and apply focused, consistent action to address them.

The M3 Recap

- **Metabolic dysfunction** leads to visceral fat accumulation, abnormal blood sugar control, abnormal cholesterol profiles, and high blood pressure. These are the core ingredients of metabolic syndrome and the early seeds of cardiovascular disease.
- **Malignancy**, or the development of cancer, is promoted by the same environment: insulin and IGF-1 act as growth factors, inflammation encourages mutations, and excess fat tissue alters hormone levels and immune function.
- **Memory loss**, particularly Alzheimer's and vascular dementia, shares these same risks. High blood pressure, insulin resistance, and inflammation damage small vessels in the brain and impair glucose metabolism in neurons.

You could treat each of these downstream diseases separately, or you could go upstream and address the shared cause.

The diseases most feared today, heart attacks, strokes, cancers, and dementia, are not random. They are complex but not mysterious. They are often late outcomes of early, silent processes that can be influenced years in advance.

The same strategy that prevents one often helps prevent them all. That's the core idea of the M3 framework.

The earlier you act, the better your chances. But it's never too late to start.

If you've read this far, you already have the most important thing: awareness. Now it's about action. Diet, exercise, know your numbers, establish with a primary care doctor and have all the age-appropriate screening tests up to date.

Your health isn't just about managing disease. It's about understanding how your body works and taking ownership of the most modifiable risks.

That's the M3 complex of diseases: One cause, many consequences, and one path to prevent them.

References

Abete I, Romaguera D, Vieira AR, Lopez de Munain A, Norat T. Association between total, processed, red and white meat consumption and all-cause, CVD and IHD mortality: a meta-analysis of cohort studies. Br J Nutr. 2014 Sep 14;112(5):762-75. doi: 10.1017/S000711451400124X. Epub 2014 Jun 16. PMID: 24932617.

Acosta RD, Cash BD. Clinical effects of colonic cleansing for general health promotion: a systematic review. Am J Gastroenterol. 2009 Nov;104(11):2830-6; quiz 2837. doi: 10.1038/ajg.2009.494. Epub 2009 Sep 1. Erratum in: Am J Gastroenterol. 2010 May;105(5):1214. PMID: 19724266.

American Cancer Society, ACS released Cancer Statistics, 2025. Accessed on 06/15/2025 at https://pressroom.cancer.org/2025CancerFactsandFigures

American Cancer Society, Colorectal Cancer Facts and Figures 2023-2025 accessed on 05/12/2025 at https://www.cancer.org/content/dam/cancer-org/research/cancer-facts-and-statistics/colorectal-cancer-facts-and-figures/colorectal-cancer-facts-and-figures-2023.pdf

Ashruf OS, Hundal J, Mushtaq A, Kaelber DC, Anwer F, Singh A. Hematologic Cancers Among Patients With Type 2 Diabetes Prescribed GLP-1 Receptor Agonists. JAMA Netw Open. 2025 Mar 3;8(3):e250802. doi: 10.1001/jamanetworkopen.2025.0802. PMID: 40048168; PMCID: PMC11886721.

Avadhani R, Fowler K, Barbato C, Thomas S, Wong W, Paul C, Aksakal M, Hauser TH, Weinger K, Goldfine AB Glycemia and cognitive function in metabolic syndrome and coronary heart disease. Am J Med. 2015 Jan;128(1):46-55. Epub 2014 Sep 16. PMID 25220612

Bailey CJ. Metformin: historical overview. Diabetologia. 2017 Sep;60(9):1566-1576. doi: 10.1007/s00125-017-4318-z. Epub 2017 Aug 3. PMID: 28776081.

Banach M, Serban C, Sahebkar A, Ursoniu S, Rysz J, Muntner P, Toth PP, Jones SR, Rizzo M, Glasser SP, Lip GY, Dragan S, Mikhailidis DP; Lipid and Blood Pressure Meta-analysis Collaboration Group. Effects of coenzyme Q10 on statin-induced myopathy: a meta-analysis of randomized controlled trials. Mayo Clin Proc. 2015 Jan;90(1):24-34. doi: 10.1016/j.mayocp.2014.08.021. Epub 2014 Nov 14. PMID: 25440725.

Barnard ND, Katcher HI, Jenkins DJ, Cohen J, Turner-McGrievy G. Vegetarian and vegan diets in type 2 diabetes management. Nutr Rev. 2009 May;67(5):255-63. doi: 10.1111/j.1753-4887.2009.00198.x. PMID: 19386029.

Barry VW, Baruth M, Beets MW, Durstine JL, Liu J, Blair SN. Fitness vs. fatness on all-cause mortality: a meta-analysis. Prog Cardiovasc Dis. 2014 Jan-Feb;56(4):382-90. doi: 10.1016/j.pcad.2013.09.002. Epub 2013 Oct 11. PMID: 24438729.

Bartke, A. (2008). "Impact of reduced insulin-like growth factor-1/insulin signaling on aging in mammals." Cell Metabolism.

Biddle KD, d'Oleire Uquillas F, Jacobs HIL, Zide B, Kirn DR, Rentz DM, Johnson KA, Sperling RA, Donovan NJ. Social Engagement and Amyloid-β-Related Cognitive Decline in Cognitively Normal Older Adults. Am J Geriatr Psychiatry. 2019 Nov;27(11):1247-1256. doi: 10.1016/j.jagp.2019.05.005. Epub 2019 May 10. PMID: 31248770; PMCID: PMC6778491.

Blackburn, E. H., Epel, E. S., & Lin, J. (2015). "Telomeres and aging-related diseases." New England Journal of Medicine.

Brunchmann A, Thomsen M, Fink-Jensen A. The effect of glucagon-like peptide-1 (GLP-1) receptor agonists on substance use disorder (SUD)-related behavioural effects of drugs and alcohol: A systematic review. Physiol Behav. 2019 Jul 1;206:232-242. doi: 10.1016/j.physbeh.2019.03.029. Epub 2019 Apr 1. PMID: 30946836; PMCID: PMC6520118.

Burke AP, Farb A, Malcom GT, Liang Y, Smialek JE, Virmani R. Plaque rupture and sudden death related to exertion in men with coronary artery disease.

JAMA. 1999 Mar 10;281(10):921-6. doi: 10.1001/jama.281.10.921. PMID: 10078489.

de Cabo R, Mattson MP. Effects of Intermittent Fasting on Health, Aging, and Disease. N Engl J Med. 2019 Dec 26;381(26):2541-2551. doi: 10.1056/NEJMra1905136. Erratum in: N Engl J Med. 2020 Jan 16;382(3):298. doi: 10.1056/NEJMx190038. Erratum in: N Engl J Med. 2020 Mar 5;382(10):978. doi: 10.1056/NEJMx200002. PMID: 31881139.

Cahill K, Stevens S, Perera R, Lancaster T. Pharmacological interventions for smoking cessation: an overview and network meta-analysis. Cochrane Database Syst Rev. 2013 May 31;2013(5):CD009329. doi: 10.1002/14651858.CD009329.pub2. PMID: 23728690; PMCID: PMC8406789.

Centers for Disease Control and Prevention, Leading Causes of Death accessed on 05/15/2025 at https://www.cdc.gov/nchs/fastats/leading-causes-of-death.htm

Centers for Disease Control and Prevention, exercise recommendations accessed on 4/19/25 at https://www.cdc.gov/physical-activity-basics/guidelines/adults.html?utm_source=chatgpt.com

Centers for Disease Control and Prevention, Adult Immunization by Age, accessed on 05/12/2025 at https://www.cdc.gov/vaccines/hcp/imz-schedules/adult-age.html

Centers for Disease Control and Prevention, Child and Adolescent Immunization Schedule by Age, accessed on 05/12/2025 at https://www.cdc.gov/vaccines/hcp/imz-schedules/child-adolescent-age.html

Centers for Disease Control and Prevention, 2020 U.S. Department of Health and Human Services. Smoking Cessation: A Report of the Surgeon General. Atlanta, GA: U.S. Department of Health and Human Services, Centers for Disease Control and Prevention, National Center for Chronic Disease Prevention and Health Promotion, Office on Smoking and Health, 2020, accessed on 04/24/2025 at https://www.hhs.gov/sites/default/files/2020-cessation-sgr-full-report.pdf

Centers for Disease Control and Prevention, About Sleep, accessed on 5/18/2025 at https://www.cdc.gov/sleep/about/index.html

Chetty, R., Stepner, M., Abraham, S., et al. (2016). "The Association Between Income and Life Expectancy in the United States, 2001-2014." JAMA.

Cholesterol Treatment Trialists' Collaboration. (2019). "Efficacy and safety of statin therapy in older people: A meta-analysis of individual participant data from 28 randomised controlled trials." The Lancet.

Choi J, Nguyen VH, Przybyszewski E, Song J, Carroll A, Michta M, Almazan E, Simon TG, Chung RT. Statin Use and Risk of Hepatocellular Carcinoma and Liver Fibrosis in Chronic Liver Disease. JAMA Intern Med. 2025 May 1;185(5):522-530. doi: 10.1001/jamainternmed.2025.0115. PMID: 40094696; PMCID: PMC11915111.

Collaborative Group on Hormonal Factors in Breast Cancer, Breast cancer and hormone replacement therapy: collaborative reanalysis of data from 51 epidemiological studies of 52,705 women with breast cancer and 108,411 women without breast cancer. Lancet. 1997 Oct 11;350(9084):1047-59. Erratum in: Lancet 1997 Nov 15;350(9089):1484. PMID: 10213546.

Collins R, Reith C, Emberson J, Armitage J, Baigent C, Blackwell L, Blumenthal R, Danesh J, Smith GD, DeMets D, Evans S, Law M, MacMahon S, Martin S, Neal B, Poulter N, Preiss D, Ridker P, Roberts I, Rodgers A, Sandercock P, Schulz K, Sever P, Simes J, Smeeth L, Wald N, Yusuf S, Peto R. Interpretation of the evidence for the efficacy and safety of statin therapy. Lancet. 2016 Nov 19;388(10059):2532-2561. doi: 10.1016/S0140-6736(16)31357-5. Epub 2016 Sep 8. Erratum in: Lancet 2017 Feb 11;389(10069):602. doi: 10.1016/S0140-6736(16)31468-4. PMID: 27616593.

Consensus Conference Panel; Watson NF, Badr MS, Belenky G, Bliwise DL, Buxton OM, Buysse D, Dinges DF, Gangwisch J, Grandner MA, Kushida C, Malhotra RK, Martin JL, Patel SR, Quan SF, Tasali E; Non-Participating Observers; Twery M, Croft JB, Maher E; American Academy of Sleep Medicine Staff; Barrett JA, Thomas SM, Heald JL. Recommended Amount of Sleep for a

Healthy Adult: A Joint Consensus Statement of the American Academy of Sleep Medicine and Sleep Research Society. J Clin Sleep Med. 2015 Jun 15;11(6):591-2. doi: 10.5664/jcsm.4758. PMID: 25979105; PMCID: PMC4442216.

Criqui MH, Denenberg JO, Ix JH, McClelland RL, Wassel CL, Rifkin DE, Carr JJ, Budoff MJ, Allison MA. Calcium density of coronary artery plaque and risk of incident cardiovascular events. JAMA. 2014 Jan 15;311(3):271-8. doi: 10.1001/jama.2013.282535. Erratum in: JAMA. 2015 Apr 7;313(13):1374. doi: 10.1001/jama.2014.16845. PMID: 24247483; PMCID: PMC4091626.

Crowley R, Daniel H, Cooney TG, et al; for the Health and Public Policy Committee of the American College of Physicians. Envisioning a Better U.S. Health Care System for All: Coverage and Cost of Care. Ann Intern Med.2020;172:S7-S32. [Epub 21 January 2020]. doi:10.7326/M19-2415

Cutler, D. M., & Miller, G. (2005). "The role of public health improvements in health advances." Proceedings of the National Academy of Sciences.

Delgado-Lista J, Alcala-Diaz JF, Torres-Peña JD, Quintana-Navarro GM, Fuentes F, Garcia-Rios A, Ortiz-Morales AM, Gonzalez-Requero AI, Perez-Caballero AI, Yubero-Serrano EM, Rangel-Zuñiga OA, Camargo A, Rodriguez-Cantalejo F, Lopez-Segura F, Badimon L, Ordovas JM, Perez-Jimenez F, Perez-Martinez P, Lopez-Miranda J; CORDIOPREV Investigators. Long-term secondary prevention of cardiovascular disease with a Mediterranean diet and a low-fat diet (CORDIOPREV): a randomised controlled trial. Lancet. 2022 May 14;399(10338):1876-1885. doi: 10.1016/S0140-6736(22)00122-2. Epub 2022 May 4. PMID: 35525255.

Durham DD, Abraham LA, Roberts MC, Khan CP, Smith RA, Kerlikowske K, Miglioretti DL. Breast cancer incidence among women with a family history of breast cancer by relative's age at diagnosis. Cancer. 2022 Dec 15;128(24):4232-4240. doi: 10.1002/cncr.34365. Epub 2022 Oct 19. PMID: 36262035; PMCID: PMC9712500.

Egan BM, Lackland DT, Sutherland SE, Rakotz MK, Williams J, Commodore-Mensah Y, Jones DW, Kjeldsen SE, Campbell NRC, Parati G, He FJ, MacGregor

GA, Weber MA, Whelton PK. PERSPECTIVE - The Growing Global Benefits of Limiting Salt Intake: an urgent call from the World Hypertension League for more effective policy and public health initiatives. J Hum Hypertens. 2025 Apr;39(4):241-245. doi: 10.1038/s41371-025-00990-1. Epub 2025 Mar 21. PMID: 40119141; PMCID: PMC11985337.

Ettehad D, Emdin CA, Kiran A, Anderson SG, Callender T, Emberson J, Chalmers J, Rodgers A, Rahimi K. Blood pressure lowering for prevention of cardiovascular disease and death: a systematic review and meta-analysis. Lancet. 2016 Mar 5;387(10022):957-967. doi: 10.1016/S0140-6736(15)01225-8. Epub 2015 Dec 24. PMID: 26724178.

Faksova K, Walsh D, Jiang Y, Griffin J, Phillips A, Gentile A, Kwong JC, Macartney K, Naus M, Grange Z, Escolano S, Sepulveda G, Shetty A, Pillsbury A, Sullivan C, Naveed Z, Janjua NZ, Giglio N, Perälä J, Nasreen S, Gidding H, Hovi P, Vo T, Cui F, Deng L, Cullen L, Artama M, Lu H, Clothier HJ, Batty K, Paynter J, Petousis-Harris H, Buttery J, Black S, Hviid A. COVID-19 vaccines and adverse events of special interest: A multinational Global Vaccine Data Network (GVDN) cohort study of 99 million vaccinated individuals. Vaccine. 2024 Apr 2;42(9):2200-2211. doi: 10.1016/j.vaccine.2024.01.100. Epub 2024 Feb 12. PMID: 38350768.

Ference BA, Ginsberg HN, Graham I, Ray KK, Packard CJ, Bruckert E, Hegele RA, Krauss RM, Raal FJ, Schunkert H, Watts GF, Borén J, Fazio S, Horton JD, Masana L, Nicholls SJ, Nordestgaard BG, van de Sluis B, Taskinen MR, Tokgözoglu L, Landmesser U, Laufs U, Wiklund O, Stock JK, Chapman MJ, Catapano AL. Low-density lipoproteins cause atherosclerotic cardiovascular disease. 1. Evidence from genetic, epidemiologic, and clinical studies. A consensus statement from the European Atherosclerosis Society Consensus Panel. Eur Heart J. 2017 Aug 21;38(32):2459-2472. doi: 10.1093/eurheartj/ehx144. PMID: 28444290; PMCID: PMC5837225.

Ferencik M, Chatzizisis YS. Statins and the coronary plaque calcium "paradox": Insights from non-invasive and invasive imaging. Atherosclerosis. 2015

Aug;241(2):783-5. doi: 10.1016/j.atherosclerosis.2015.05.021. Epub 2015 Jun 3. PMID: 26070488.

Feskens EJ, Sluik D, van Woudenbergh GJ. Meat consumption, diabetes, and its complications. Curr Diab Rep. 2013 Apr;13(2):298-306. doi: 10.1007/s11892-013-0365-0. PMID: 23354681.

Fontana L, Partridge L, Longo VD. Extending healthy life span--from yeast to humans. Science. 2010 Apr 16;328(5976):321-6. doi: 10.1126/science.1172539. PMID: 20395504; PMCID: PMC3607354.

Frontera JA, Tamborska AA, Doheim MF, Garcia-Azorin D, Gezegen H, Guekht A, Yusof Khan AHK, Santacatterina M, Sejvar J, Thakur KT, Westenberg E, Winkler AS, Beghi E; contributors from the Global COVID-19 Neuro Research Coalition. Neurological Events Reported after COVID-19 Vaccines: An Analysis of VAERS. Ann Neurol. 2022 Mar 2;91(6):756–71. doi: 10.1002/ana.26339. Epub ahead of print. PMID: 35233819; PMCID: PMC9082459.

Gallagher EJ, LeRoith D. Obesity and Diabetes: The Increased Risk of Cancer and Cancer-Related Mortality. Physiol Rev. 2015 Jul;95(3):727-48. doi: 10.1152/physrev.00030.2014. PMID: 26084689; PMCID: PMC4491542.

Garcia L, Pearce M, Abbas A, Mok A, Strain T, Ali S, Crippa A, Dempsey PC, Golubic R, Kelly P, Laird Y, McNamara E, Moore S, de Sa TH, Smith AD, Wijndaele K, Woodcock J, Brage S. Non-occupational physical activity and risk of cardiovascular disease, cancer and mortality outcomes: a dose-response meta-analysis of large prospective studies. Br J Sports Med. 2023 Aug;57(15):979-989. doi: 10.1136/bjsports-2022-105669. Epub 2023 Feb 28. PMID: 36854652; PMCID: PMC10423495.

Giugliano, D., Scappaticcio, L., Longo, M. et al. GLP-1 receptor agonists and cardiorenal outcomes in type 2 diabetes: an updated meta-analysis of eight CVOTs. Cardiovasc Diabetol 20, 189 (2021). https://doi.org/10.1186/s12933-021-01366-8

Gottesman RF, Albert MS, Alonso A, Coker LH, Coresh J, Davis SM, Deal JA, McKhann GM, Mosley TH, Sharrett AR, Schneider ALC, Windham BG, Wruck

LM, Knopman DS, Associations Between Midlife Vascular Risk Factors and 25-Year Incident Dementia in the Atherosclerosis Risk in Communities (ARIC) Cohort. JAMA Neurol. 2017;74(10):1246 PMID 28783817

Grossman E, Messerli FH. Long-term safety of antihypertensive therapy. Prog Cardiovasc Dis. 2006 Jul-Aug;49(1):16-25. doi: 10.1016/j.pcad.2006.06.002. PMID: 16867847.

Guyton and Hall, Textbook of Medical Physiology, Fourteenth Edition, Elsevier, 2021, p.886

Haskell WL, Lee IM, Pate RR, Powell KE, Blair SN, Franklin BA, Macera CA, Heath GW, Thompson PD, Bauman A; American College of Sports Medicine; American Heart Association. Physical activity and public health: updated recommendation for adults from the American College of Sports Medicine and the American Heart Association. Circulation. 2007 Aug 28;116(9):1081-93. doi: 10.1161/CIRCULATIONAHA.107.185649. Epub 2007 Aug 1. PMID: 17671237.

He FJ, MacGregor GA. A comprehensive review on salt and health and current experience of worldwide salt reduction programmes. J Hum Hypertens. 2009 Jun;23(6):363-84. doi: 10.1038/jhh.2008.144. Epub 2008 Dec 25. PMID: 19110538.

Holt-Lunstad J, Smith TB, Layton JB. Social relationships and mortality risk: a meta-analytic review. PLoS Med. 2010 Jul 27;7(7):e1000316. doi: 10.1371/journal.pmed.1000316. PMID: 20668659; PMCID: PMC2910600.

Howard JP, Wood FA, Finegold JA, Nowbar AN, Thompson DM, Arnold AD, Rajkumar CA, Connolly S, Cegla J, Stride C, Sever P, Norton C, Thom SAM, Shun-Shin MJ, Francis DP. Side Effect Patterns in a Crossover Trial of Statin, Placebo, and No Treatment. J Am Coll Cardiol. 2021 Sep 21;78(12):1210-1222. doi: 10.1016/j.jacc.2021.07.022. PMID: 34531021; PMCID: PMC8453640.

Htike ZZ, Zaccardi F, Papamargaritis D, Webb DR, Khunti K, Davies MJ. Efficacy and safety of glucagon-like peptide-1 receptor agonists in type 2 diabetes: A systematic review and mixed-treatment comparison analysis.

Diabetes Obes Metab. 2017 Apr;19(4):524-536. doi: 10.1111/dom.12849. Epub 2017 Feb 17. PMID: 27981757.

Huang YN, Liao WL, Huang JY, Lin YJ, Yang SF, Huang CC, Wang CH, Su PH. Long-term safety and efficacy of glucagon-like peptide-1 receptor agonists in individuals with obesity and without type 2 diabetes: A global retrospective cohort study. Diabetes Obes Metab. 2024 Nov;26(11):5222-5232. doi: 10.1111/dom.15869. Epub 2024 Aug 22. Erratum in: Diabetes Obes Metab. 2025 Mar;27(3):1630. doi: 10.1111/dom.16204. PMID: 39171569.

Huesch, D., and Mosher, T. J. (2017). Using It or Losing It? The Case for Data Scientists Inside Health Care. NeJM Catalyst. Available online at: https://catalyst.nejm.org/case-data-scientists-inside-health-care/

Inoue K, Tsugawa Y, Mayeda ER, Ritz B. Association of Daily Step Patterns With Mortality in US Adults. JAMA Netw Open. 2023;6(3):e235174. doi:10.1001/jamanetworkopen.2023.5174

Inoue M, Yamamoto S, Kurahashi N, Iwasaki M, Sasazuki S, Tsugane S; Japan Public Health Center-based Prospective Study Group. Daily total physical activity level and total cancer risk in men and women: results from a large-scale population-based cohort study in Japan. Am J Epidemiol. 2008 Aug 15;168(4):391-403. doi: 10.1093/aje/kwn146. Epub 2008 Jul 2. PMID: 18599492.

Jerlhag E. GLP-1 Receptor Agonists: Promising Therapeutic Targets for Alcohol Use Disorder. Endocrinology. 2025 Feb 27;166(4):bqaf028. doi: 10.1210/endocr/bqaf028. PMID: 39980336; PMCID: PMC11879929.

Jeong SM, Choi S, Kim K, Kim SM, Lee G, Park SY, Kim YY, Son JS, Yun JM, Park SM. Effect of Change in Total Cholesterol Levels on Cardiovascular Disease Among Young Adults. J Am Heart Assoc. 2018 Jun 13;7(12):e008819. doi: 10.1161/JAHA.118.008819. PMID: 29899019; PMCID: PMC6220545.

Jick H, Zornberg GL, Jick SS, Seshadri S, Drachman DA. Statins and the risk of dementia. Lancet. 2000 Nov 11;356(9242):1627-31. doi: 10.1016/s0140-6736(00)03155-x. Erratum in: Lancet 2001 Feb 17;357(9255):562. PMID: 11089820.

Jones PH, Davidson MH, Stein EA, Bays HE, McKenney JM, Miller E, Cain VA, Blasetto JW; STELLAR Study Group. Comparison of the efficacy and safety of rosuvastatin versus atorvastatin, simvastatin, and pravastatin across doses (STELLAR* Trial). Am J Cardiol. 2003 Jul 15;92(2):152-60. doi: 10.1016/s0002-9149(03)00530-7. PMID: 12860216.

Jung E, Kong SY, Ro YS, Ryu HH, Shin SD. Serum Cholesterol Levels and Risk of Cardiovascular Death: A Systematic Review and a Dose-Response Meta-Analysis of Prospective Cohort Studies. Int J Environ Res Public Health. 2022 Jul 6;19(14):8272. doi: 10.3390/ijerph19148272. PMID: 35886124; PMCID: PMC9316578.

Kaluza J, Wolk A, Larsson SC. Red meat consumption and risk of stroke: a meta-analysis of prospective studies. Stroke. 2012 Oct;43(10):2556-60. doi: 10.1161/STROKEAHA.112.663286. Epub 2012 Jul 31. PMID: 22851546.

Kaner EF, Beyer F, Dickinson HO, Pienaar E, Campbell F, Schlesinger C, Heather N, Saunders J, Burnand B. Effectiveness of brief alcohol interventions in primary care populations. Cochrane Database Syst Rev. 2007 Apr 18;(2):CD004148. doi: 10.1002/14651858.CD004148.pub3. Update in: Cochrane Database Syst Rev. 2018 Feb 24;2:CD004148. doi: 10.1002/14651858.CD004148.pub4. PMID: 17443541.

Karam G, Agarwal A, Sadeghirad B, Jalink M, Hitchcock CL, Ge L, Kiflen R, Ahmed W, Zea AM, Milenkovic J, Chedrawe MA, Rabassa M, El Dib R, Goldenberg JZ, Guyatt GH, Boyce E, Johnston BC. Comparison of seven popular structured dietary programmes and risk of mortality and major cardiovascular events in patients at increased cardiovascular risk: systematic review and network meta-analysis. BMJ. 2023 Mar 29;380:e072003. doi: 10.1136/bmj-2022-072003. PMID: 36990505; PMCID: PMC10053756.

Kenyon, C. The genetics of ageing. *Nature* 464, 504–512 (2010). https://doi.org/10.1038/nature08980

Khan SU, Yedlapati SH, Lone AN, Hao Q, Guyatt G, Delvaux N, Bekkering GET, Vandvik PO, Riaz IB, Li S, Aertgeerts B, Rodondi N. PCSK9 inhibitors and ezetimibe with or without statin therapy for cardiovascular risk reduction: a systematic review and network meta-analysis. BMJ. 2022 May 4;377:e069116. doi: 10.1136/bmj-2021-069116. PMID: 35508321.

King, A. Health risks of physical inactivity similar to smoking. Nat Rev Cardiol 9, 492 (2012). https://doi.org/10.1038/nrcardio.2012.115

Knowler WC, Barrett-Connor E, Fowler SE, Hamman RF, Lachin JM, Walker EA, Nathan DM; Diabetes Prevention Program Research Group. Reduction in the incidence of type 2 diabetes with lifestyle intervention or metformin. N Engl J Med. 2002 Feb 7;346(6):393-403. doi: 10.1056/NEJMoa012512. PMID: 11832527; PMCID: PMC1370926.

Kosiborod MN, Abildstrøm SZ, Borlaug BA, Butler J, Rasmussen S, Davies M, Hovingh GK, Kitzman DW, Lindegaard ML, Møller DV, Shah SJ, Treppendahl MB, Verma S, Abhayaratna W, Ahmed FZ, Chopra V, Ezekowitz J, Fu M, Ito H, Lelonek M, Melenovsky V, Merkely B, Núñez J, Perna E, Schou M, Senni M, Sharma K, Van der Meer P, von Lewinski D, Wolf D, Petrie MC; STEP-HFpEF Trial Committees and Investigators. Semaglutide in Patients with Heart Failure with Preserved Ejection Fraction and Obesity. N Engl J Med. 2023 Sep 21;389(12):1069-1084. doi: 10.1056/NEJMoa2306963. Epub 2023 Aug 25. PMID: 37622681.

Kratzer TB, Siegel RL, Miller KD, Sung H, Islami F, Jemal A. Progress Against Cancer Mortality 50 Years After Passage of the National Cancer Act. JAMA Oncol. 2022;8(1):156–159. doi:10.1001/jamaoncol.2021.5668

Kreidieh M, Hamadi R, Alsheikh M, Al Moussawi H, Deeb L. Statin Use in Patients With Chronic Liver Disease and Cirrhosis: Current Evidence and Future Directions. Gastroenterology Res. 2022 Feb;15(1):1-12. doi: 10.14740/gr1498. Epub 2022 Feb 25. PMID: 35369681; PMCID: PMC8913022.

Krueger KR, Wilson RS, Kamenetsky JM, Barnes LL, Bienias JL, Bennett DA. Social engagement and cognitive function in old age. Exp Aging Res. 2009 Jan-Mar;35(1):45-60. doi:10.1080/03610730802545028. PMID: 19173101; PMCID: PMC2758920.

Lardizabal JA, Deedwania PC. Benefits of statin therapy and compliance in high risk cardiovascular patients. Vasc Health Risk Manag. 2010 Oct 5;6:843-53. doi: 10.2147/VHRM.S9474. PMID: 20957130; PMCID: PMC2952453.

Lawes CM, Bennett DA, Feigin VL, Rodgers A. Blood pressure and stroke: an overview of published reviews. Stroke. 2004 Mar;35(3):776-85. doi: 10.1161/01.STR.0000116869.64771.5A. Epub 2004 Feb 19. Corrected and republished in: Stroke. 2004 Apr;35(4):1024. PMID: 14976329.

Leitzmann MF, Park Y, Blair A, Ballard-Barbash R, Mouw T, Hollenbeck AR, Schatzkin A. Physical activity recommendations and decreased risk of mortality. Arch Intern Med. 2007 Dec 10;167(22):2453-60. doi: 10.1001/archinte.167.22.2453. PMID: 18071167.

Lennon MJ, Lam BCP, Lipnicki DM, Crawford JD, Peters R, Schutte AE, Brodaty H, Thalamuthu A, Rydberg-Sterner T, Najar J, Skoog I, Riedel-Heller SG, Röhr S, Pabst A, Lobo A, De-la-Cámara C, Lobo E, Bello T, Gureje O, Ojagbemi A, Lipton RB, Katz MJ, Derby CA, Kim KW, Han JW, Oh DJ, Rolandi E, Davin A, Rossi M, Scarmeas N, Yannakoulia M, Dardiotis T, Hendrie HC, Gao S, Carrière I, Ritchie K, Anstey KJ, Cherbuin N, Xiao S, Yue L, Li W, Guerchet MM, Preux PM, Aboyans V, Haan MN, Aiello AE, Ng TP, Nyunt MSZ, Gao Q, Scazufca M, Sachdev PSS. Use of Antihypertensives, Blood Pressure, and Estimated Risk of Dementia in Late Life: An Individual Participant Data Meta-Analysis. JAMA Netw Open. 2023 Sep 5;6(9):e2333353. doi: 10.1001/jamanetworkopen.2023.33353. PMID: 37698858; PMCID: PMC10498335.

Levy S, Attia A, Elshazli RM, Abdelmaksoud A, Tatum D, Aiash H, Toraih EA. Differential Effects of GLP-1 Receptor Agonists on Cancer Risk in Obesity: A Nationwide Analysis of 1.1 Million Patients. Cancers (Basel). 2024 Dec 30;17(1):78. doi: 10.3390/cancers17010078. PMID: 39796706; PMCID: PMC11720624.

Li G, Shofer JB, Rhew IC, Kukull WA, Peskind ER, McCormick W, Bowen JD, Schellenberg GD, Crane PK, Breitner JC, Larson EB. Age-varying association between statin use and incident Alzheimer's disease. J Am Geriatr Soc. 2010

Jul;58(7):1311-7. doi: 10.1111/j.1532-5415.2010.02906.x. Epub 2010 Jun 1. PMID: 20533968; PMCID: PMC3176730.

Li M, Lin H, Yang Q, Zhang X, Zhou Q, Shi J, Ge F. Glucagon-like peptide-1 receptor agonists for the treatment of obstructive sleep apnea: a meta-analysis. Sleep. 2025 Apr 11;48(4):zsae280. doi: 10.1093/sleep/zsae280. PMID: 39626095.

Li S, Stampfer MJ, Williams DR, VanderWeele TJ. Association of Religious Service Attendance With Mortality Among Women. JAMA Intern Med. 2016 Jun 1;176(6):777-85. doi: 10.1001/jamainternmed.2016.1615. PMID: 27183175; PMCID: PMC5503841.

Lincoff AM, Brown-Frandsen K, Colhoun HM, Deanfield J, Emerson SS, Esbjerg S, Hardt-Lindberg S, Hovingh GK, Kahn SE, Kushner RF, Lingvay I, Oral TK, Michelsen MM, Plutzky J, Tornøe CW, Ryan DH; SELECT Trial Investigators. Semaglutide and Cardiovascular Outcomes in Obesity without Diabetes. N Engl J Med. 2023 Dec 14;389(24):2221-2232. doi: 10.1056/NEJMoa2307563. Epub 2023 Nov 11. PMID: 37952131.

Livingston G, Sommerlad A, Orgeta V, Costafreda SG, Huntley J, Ames D, Ballard C, Banerjee S, Burns A, Cohen-Mansfield J, Cooper C, Fox N, Gitlin LN, Howard R, Kales HC, Larson EB, Ritchie K, Rockwood K, Sampson EL, Samus Q, Schneider LS, Selbæk G, Teri L, Mukadam N Dementia prevention, intervention, and care. Lancet. 2017;390(10113):2673. Epub 2017 Jul 20. PMID 28735855

Loomba R, Hartman ML, Lawitz EJ, Vuppalanchi R, Boursier J, Bugianesi E, Yoneda M, Behling C, Cummings OW, Tang Y, Brouwers B, Robins DA, Nikooie A, Bunck MC, Haupt A, Sanyal AJ; SYNERGY-NASH Investigators. Tirzepatide for Metabolic Dysfunction-Associated Steatohepatitis with Liver Fibrosis. N Engl J Med. 2024 Jul 25;391(4):299-310. doi: 10.1056/NEJMoa2401943. Epub 2024 Jun 8. PMID: 38856224.

Lord JM, Flight IH, Norman RJ. Metformin in polycystic ovary syndrome: systematic review and meta-analysis. BMJ. 2003 Oct 25;327(7421):951-3. doi: 10.1136/bmj.327.7421.951. PMID: 14576245; PMCID: PMC259161

Loy CT, Schofield PR, Turner AM, Kwok JB. Genetics of dementia. Lancet. 2014 Mar 1;383(9919):828-40. doi: 10.1016/S0140-6736(13)60630-3. Epub 2013 Aug 6. PMID: 23927914.

Luchsinger JA, Reitz C, Honig LS, Tang MX, Shea S, Mayeux R Aggregation of vascular risk factors and risk of incident Alzheimer disease. Neurology. 2005;65(4):545. PMID 16116114

Luna-Marco C, de Marañon AM, Hermo-Argibay A, Rodriguez-Hernandez Y, Hermenejildo J, Fernandez-Reyes M, Apostolova N, Vila J, Sola E, Morillas C, Rovira-Llopis S, Rocha M, Victor VM. Effects of GLP-1 receptor agonists on mitochondrial function, inflammatory markers and leukocyte-endothelium interactions in type 2 diabetes. Redox Biol. 2023 Oct;66:102849. doi: 10.1016/j.redox.2023.102849. Epub 2023 Aug 14. PMID: 37591012; PMCID: PMC10457591.

Magnan, S. 2017. Social Determinants of Health 101 for Health Care: Five Plus Five. *NAM Perspectives*. Discussion Paper, National Academy of Medicine, Washington, DC. https://doi.org/10.31478/201710c

Mandsager K, Harb S, Cremer P, Phelan D, Nissen SE, Jaber W. Association of Cardiorespiratory Fitness With Long-term Mortality Among Adults Undergoing Exercise Treadmill Testing. JAMA Netw Open. 2018;1(6):e183605. doi:10.1001/jamanetworkopen.2018.3605

Matthews T, Rasmussen LJH, Ambler A, Danese A, Eugen-Olsen J, Fancourt D, Fisher HL, Iversen KK, Schultz M, Sugden K, Williams B, Caspi A, Moffitt TE. Social isolation, loneliness, and inflammation: A multi-cohort investigation in early and mid-adulthood. Brain Behav Immun. 2024 Jan;115:727-736. doi: 10.1016/j.bbi.2023.11.022. Epub 2023 Nov 21. PMID: 37992788; PMCID: PMC11194667.

Mattson MP, Moehl K, Ghena N, Schmaedick M, Cheng A. Intermittent metabolic switching, neuroplasticity and brain health. Nat Rev Neurosci. 2018 Feb;19(2):63-80. doi: 10.1038/nrn.2017.156. Epub 2018 Jan 11. Erratum in: Nat

Rev Neurosci. 2020 Aug;21(8):445. doi: 10.1038/s41583-020-0342-y. PMID: 29321682; PMCID: PMC5913738.

Mattson MP, Arumugam TV. Hallmarks of Brain Aging: Adaptive and Pathological Modification by Metabolic States. Cell Metab. 2018 Jun 5;27(6):1176-1199. doi: 10.1016/j.cmet.2018.05.011. PMID: 29874566; PMCID: PMC6039826.

McTiernan A, Friedenreich CM, Katzmarzyk PT, Powell KE, Macko R, Buchner D, Pescatello LS, Bloodgood B, Tennant B, Vaux-Bjerke A, George SM, Troiano RP, Piercy KL; 2018 PHYSICAL ACTIVITY GUIDELINES ADVISORY COMMITTEE*. Physical Activity in Cancer Prevention and Survival: A Systematic Review. Med Sci Sports Exerc. 2019 Jun;51(6):1252-1261. doi: 10.1249/MSS.0000000000001937. PMID: 31095082; PMCID: PMC6527123.

Monzio Compagnoni, G., Di Fonzo, A., Corti, S. et al. The Role of Mitochondria in Neurodegenerative Diseases: the Lesson from Alzheimer's Disease and Parkinson's Disease. Mol Neurobiol 57, 2959–2980 (2020). https://doi.org/10.1007/s12035-020-01926-1

Moore SC, Lee IM, Weiderpass E, Campbell PT, Sampson JN, Kitahara CM, Keadle SK, Arem H, Berrington de Gonzalez A, Hartge P, Adami HO, Blair CK, Borch KB, Boyd E, Check DP, Fournier A, Freedman ND, Gunter M, Johannson M, Khaw KT, Linet MS, Orsini N, Park Y, Riboli E, Robien K, Schairer C, Sesso H, Spriggs M, Van Dusen R, Wolk A, Matthews CE, Patel AV. Association of Leisure-Time Physical Activity With Risk of 26 Types of Cancer in 1.44 Million Adults. JAMA Intern Med. 2016 Jun 1;176(6):816-25. doi: 10.1001/jamainternmed.2016.1548. PMID: 27183032; PMCID: PMC5812009.

Newman CB, Preiss D, Tobert JA, Jacobson TA, Page RL 2nd, Goldstein LB, Chin C, Tannock LR, Miller M, Raghuveer G, Duell PB, Brinton EA, Pollak A, Braun LT, Welty FK; American Heart Association Clinical Lipidology, Lipoprotein, Metabolism and Thrombosis Committee, a Joint Committee of the Council on Atherosclerosis, Thrombosis and Vascular Biology and Council on Lifestyle and Cardiometabolic Health; Council on Cardiovascular Disease in the Young; Council on Clinical Cardiology; and Stroke Council. Statin Safety and

Associated Adverse Events: A Scientific Statement From the American Heart Association. Arterioscler Thromb Vasc Biol. 2019 Feb;39(2):e38-e81. doi: 10.1161/ATV.0000000000000073. Erratum in: Arterioscler Thromb Vasc Biol. 2019 May;39(5):e158. doi: 10.1161/ATV.0000000000000081. PMID: 30580575.

Nicholls SJ, Ballantyne CM, Barter PJ, Chapman MJ, Erbel RM, Libby P, Raichlen JS, Uno K, Borgman M, Wolski K, Nissen SE. Effect of two intensive statin regimens on progression of coronary disease. N Engl J Med. 2011 Dec 1;365(22):2078-87. doi: 10.1056/NEJMoa1110874. Epub 2011 Nov 15. PMID: 22085316.

National Institutes of Health, Healthy Eating Plan, accessed on 04/21/2025 at https://www.nhlbi.nih.gov/health/educational/lose_wt/eat/calories.htm?utm_source=chatgpt.com on

National Institutes of Health, What is sleep apnea, accessed on 05/18/2025 at https://www.nhlbi.nih.gov/health/sleep-apnea

Nissen SE, Nicholls SJ, Sipahi I, Libby P, Raichlen JS, Ballantyne CM, Davignon J, Erbel R, Fruchart JC, Tardif JC, Schoenhagen P, Crowe T, Cain V, Wolski K, Goormastic M, Tuzcu EM; ASTEROID Investigators. Effect of very high-intensity statin therapy on regression of coronary atherosclerosis: the ASTEROID trial. JAMA. 2006 Apr 5;295(13):1556-65. doi: 10.1001/jama.295.13.jpc60002. Epub 2006 Mar 13. PMID: 16533939.

Nordestgaard BG, Langsted A, Mora S, Kolovou G, Baum H, Bruckert E, Watts GF, Sypniewska G, Wiklund O, Borén J, Chapman MJ, Cobbaert C, Descamps OS, von Eckardstein A, Kamstrup PR, Pulkki K, Kronenberg F, Remaley AT, Rifai N, Ros E, Langlois M; European Atherosclerosis Society (EAS) and the European Federation of Clinical Chemistry and Laboratory Medicine (EFLM) joint consensus initiative. Fasting is not routinely required for determination of a lipid profile: clinical and laboratory implications including flagging at desirable concentration cut-points-a joint consensus statement from the European Atherosclerosis Society and European Federation of Clinical Chemistry and Laboratory Medicine. Eur Heart J. 2016 Jul 1;37(25):1944-58. doi:

10.1093/eurheartj/ehw152. Epub 2016 Apr 26. PMID: 27122601; PMCID: PMC4929379.

Nuamnaichati N, Mangmool S, Chattipakorn N and Parichatikanond W (2020) Stimulation of GLP-1 Receptor Inhibits Methylglyoxal-Induced Mitochondrial Dysfunctions in H9c2 Cardiomyoblasts: Potential Role of Epac/PI3K/Akt Pathway. Front. Pharmacol. 11:805. doi: 10.3389/fphar.2020.00805

Oken MM, Hocking WG, Kvale PA, Andriole GL, Buys SS, Church TR, Crawford ED, Fouad MN, Isaacs C, Reding DJ, Weissfeld JL, Yokochi LA, O'Brien B, Ragard LR, Rathmell JM, Riley TL, Wright P, Caparaso N, Hu P, Izmirlian G, Pinsky PF, Prorok PC, Kramer BS, Miller AB, Gohagan JK, Berg CD; PLCO Project Team. Screening by chest radiograph and lung cancer mortality: the Prostate, Lung, Colorectal, and Ovarian (PLCO) randomized trial. JAMA. 2011 Nov 2;306(17):1865-73. doi: 10.1001/jama.2011.1591. Epub 2011 Oct 26. PMID: 22031728.

Olshansky SJ, Ault AB. The fourth stage of the epidemiologic transition: the age of delayed degenerative diseases. Milbank Q. 1986;64(3):355-91. PMID: 3762504..

Orkaby AR, Driver JA, Ho Y, et al. Association of Statin Use With All-Cause and Cardiovascular Mortality in US Veterans 75 Years and Older. JAMA. 2020;324(1):68–78. doi:10.1001/jama.2020.7848

Orlich MJ, Singh PN, Sabaté J, Jaceldo-Siegl K, Fan J, Knutsen S, Beeson WL, Fraser GE. Vegetarian dietary patterns and mortality in Adventist Health Study 2. JAMA Intern Med. 2013 Jul 8;173(13):1230-8. doi: 10.1001/jamainternmed.2013.6473. PMID: 23836264; PMCID: PMC4191896.

Ott BR, Daiello LA, Dahabreh IJ, Springate BA, Bixby K, Murali M, Trikalinos TA. Do statins impair cognition? A systematic review and meta-analysis of randomized controlled trials. J Gen Intern Med. 2015 Mar;30(3):348-58. doi: 10.1007/s11606-014-3115-3. Epub 2015 Jan 10. PMID: 25575908; PMCID: PMC4351273.

Our World in Data, Statin use vs death rate from cardiovascular diseases, 2019, accessed on 05/15/2025 at https://ourworldindata.org/grapher/statin-use-cardiovascular-disease-death-rate

Parker M, Self-Brown SR, Rahimi A, Fang X. Longitudinal Analysis of the Relationship Between Social Isolation and Hypertension in Early Middle Adulthood. J Am Heart Assoc. 2024 May 7;13(9):e030403. doi: 10.1161/JAHA.123.030403. Epub 2024 Apr 15. PMID: 38619293; PMCID: PMC11179928.

Pasternak B, Wintzell V, Hviid A, Eliasson B, Gudbjörnsdottir S, Jonasson C, Hveem K, Svanström H, Melbye M, Ueda P. Glucagon-like peptide 1 receptor agonist use and risk of thyroid cancer: Scandinavian cohort study. BMJ. 2024 Apr 10;385:e078225. doi: 10.1136/bmj-2023-078225. PMID: 38683947; PMCID: PMC11004669.

Patel D, Ayesha IE, Monson NR, Klair N, Patel U, Saxena A, Hamid P. The Effectiveness of Metformin in Diabetes Prevention: A Systematic Review and Meta-Analysis. Cureus. 2023 Sep 28;15(9):e46108. doi: 10.7759/cureus.46108. PMID: 37900422; PMCID: PMC10611985.

Perkovic V, Tuttle KR, Rossing P, Mahaffey KW, Mann JFE, Bakris G, Baeres FMM, Idorn T, Bosch-Traberg H, Lausvig NL, Pratley R; FLOW Trial Committees and Investigators. Effects of Semaglutide on Chronic Kidney Disease in Patients with Type 2 Diabetes. N Engl J Med. 2024 Jul 11;391(2):109-121. doi: 10.1056/NEJMoa2403347. Epub 2024 May 24. PMID: 38785209.

Pothiwala P, Jain SK, Yaturu S. Metabolic syndrome and cancer. Metab Syndr Relat Disord. 2009 Aug;7(4):279-88. doi: 10.1089/met.2008.0065. PMID: 19284314; PMCID: PMC3191378.

Potter KJ, Phinney J, Kulai T, Munro V. Effects of GLP-1 receptor agonist therapy on resolution of steatohepatitis in non-alcoholic fatty liver disease: a systematic review and meta-analysis. J Can Assoc Gastroenterol. 2025 Jan 29;8(2):47-57. doi: 10.1093/jcag/gwae057. PMID: 40224572; PMCID: PMC11991874.

del Pozo Cruz B, Ahmadi M, Naismith SL, Stamatakis E. Association of Daily Step Count and Intensity With Incident Dementia in 78 430 Adults Living in the UK. JAMA Neurol. 2022;79(10):1059–1063. doi:10.1001/jamaneurol.2022.2672

Praud D, Rota M, Rehm J, Shield K, Zatoński W, Hashibe M, La Vecchia C, Boffetta P. Cancer incidence and mortality attributable to alcohol consumption. Int J Cancer. 2016 Mar 15;138(6):1380-7. doi: 10.1002/ijc.29890. Epub 2015 Oct 28. PMID: 26455822.

Qin J, Song L. Glucagon-like peptide-1 (GLP-1) receptor agonists and cardiovascular events in patients with type 2 diabetes mellitus: a meta-analysis of double-blind, randomized, placebo-controlled clinical trials. BMC Endocr Disord. 2022 May 12;22(1):125. doi: 10.1186/s12902-022-01036-0. PMID: 35546664; PMCID: PMC9097124.

Qin W, Yang J, Ni Y, Deng C, Ruan Q, Ruan J, Zhou P, Duan K. Efficacy and safety of once-weekly tirzepatide for weight management compared to placebo: An updated systematic review and meta-analysis including the latest SURMOUNT-2 trial. Endocrine. 2024 Oct;86(1):70-84. doi: 10.1007/s12020-024-03896-z. Epub 2024 Jun 8. PMID: 38850440; PMCID: PMC11445313.

Ridker PM, Danielson E, Fonseca FA, Genest J, Gotto AM Jr, Kastelein JJ, Koenig W, Libby P, Lorenzatti AJ, MacFadyen JG, Nordestgaard BG, Shepherd J, Willerson JT, Glynn RJ; JUPITER Study Group. Rosuvastatin to prevent vascular events in men and women with elevated C-reactive protein. N Engl J Med. 2008 Nov 20;359(21):2195-207. doi: 10.1056/NEJMoa0807646. Epub 2008 Nov 9. PMID: 18997196.

Ridker PM, Pradhan A, MacFadyen JG, Libby P, Glynn RJ. Cardiovascular benefits and diabetes risks of statin therapy in primary prevention: an analysis from the JUPITER trial. Lancet. 2012 Aug 11;380(9841):565-71. doi: 10.1016/S0140-6736(12)61190-8. PMID: 22883507; PMCID: PMC3774022.

Rodriguez PJ, Goodwin Cartwright BM, Gratzl S, Brar R, Baker C, Gluckman TJ, Stucky NL. Semaglutide vs Tirzepatide for Weight Loss in Adults With

Overweight or Obesity. JAMA Intern Med. 2024 Sep 1;184(9):1056-1064. doi: 10.1001/jamainternmed.2024.2525. PMID: 38976257; PMCID: PMC11231910.

Romieu I, Dossus L, Barquera S, Blottière HM, Franks PW, Gunter M, et al. Energy balance and obesity: what are the main drivers? Cancer Causes Control 2017;28(3):247–58. CrossRef PubMed

Rous B, Clarke CA, Hubbell E, Sasieni P. Assessment of the impact of multi-cancer early detection test screening intervals on late-stage cancer at diagnosis and mortality using a state-transition model. BMJ Open. 2025 May 8;15(5):e086648. doi: 10.1136/bmjopen-2024-086648. PMID: 40341158; PMCID: PMC12067829.

Rumgay H, Shield K, Charvat H, Ferrari P, Sornpaisarn B, Obot I, Islami F, Lemmens VEPP, Rehm J, Soerjomataram I. Global burden of cancer in 2020 attributable to alcohol consumption: a population-based study. Lancet Oncol. 2021 Aug;22(8):1071-1080. doi: 10.1016/S1470-2045(21)00279-5. PMID: 34270924; PMCID: PMC8324483.

Sabatine MS, Giugliano RP, Keech AC, Honarpour N, Wiviott SD, Murphy SA, Kuder JF, Wang H, Liu T, Wasserman SM, Sever PS, Pedersen TR; FOURIER Steering Committee and Investigators. Evolocumab and Clinical Outcomes in Patients with Cardiovascular Disease. N Engl J Med. 2017 May 4;376(18):1713-1722. doi: 10.1056/NEJMoa1615664. Epub 2017 Mar 17. PMID: 28304224.

Saint-Maurice PF, Troiano RP, Bassett DR, et al. Association of Daily Step Count and Step Intensity With Mortality Among US Adults. JAMA. 2020;323(12):1151–1160. doi:10.1001/jama.2020.1382

Sattar N, Lee MMY, Kristensen SL, Branch KRH, Del Prato S, Khurmi NS, Lam CSP, Lopes RD, McMurray JJV, Pratley RE, Rosenstock J, Gerstein HC. Cardiovascular, mortality, and kidney outcomes with GLP-1 receptor agonists in patients with type 2 diabetes: a systematic review and meta-analysis of randomised trials. Lancet Diabetes Endocrinol. 2021 Oct;9(10):653-662. doi: 10.1016/S2213-8587(21)00203-5. Epub 2021 Aug 20. PMID: 34425083.

Schmieder RE, Wassmann S, Predel HG, Weisser B, Blettenberg J, Gillessen A, Randerath O, Mevius A, Wilke T, Böhm M. Improved Persistence to Medication, Decreased Cardiovascular Events and Reduced All-Cause Mortality in Hypertensive Patients With Use of Single-Pill Combinations: Results From the START-Study. Hypertension. 2023 May;80(5):1127-1135. doi: 10.1161/HYPERTENSIONAHA.122.20810. Epub 2023 Mar 29. PMID: 36987918; PMCID: PMC10112936.

Schwingshackl L, Bogensberger B, Hoffmann G. Diet Quality as Assessed by the Healthy Eating Index, Alternate Healthy Eating Index, Dietary Approaches to Stop Hypertension Score, and Health Outcomes: An Updated Systematic Review and Meta-Analysis of Cohort Studies. J Acad Nutr Diet. 2018 Jan;118(1):74-100.e11. doi: 10.1016/j.jand.2017.08.024. Epub 2017 Oct 27. PMID: 29111090.

Schwingshackl L, Hoffmann G. Adherence to Mediterranean diet and risk of cancer: a systematic review and meta-analysis of observational studies. Int J Cancer. 2014 Oct 15;135(8):1884-97. doi: 10.1002/ijc.28824. Epub 2014 Mar 11. PMID: 24599882.

Seidelmann SB, Claggett B, Cheng S, Henglin M, Shah A, Steffen LM, Folsom AR, Rimm EB, Willett WC, Solomon SD. Dietary carbohydrate intake and mortality: a prospective cohort study and meta-analysis. Lancet Public Health. 2018 Sep;3(9):e419-e428. doi: 10.1016/S2468-2667(18)30135-X. Epub 2018 Aug 17. PMID: 30122560; PMCID: PMC6339822.

Singh BM, Lamichhane HK, Srivatsa SS, Adhikari P, Kshetri BJ, Khatiwada S, Shrestha DB. Role of Statins in the Primary Prevention of Atherosclerotic Cardiovascular Disease and Mortality in the Population with Mean Cholesterol in the Near-Optimal to Borderline High Range: A Systematic Review and Meta-Analysis. Adv Prev Med. 2020 Nov 21;2020:6617905. doi: 10.1155/2020/6617905. PMID: 33294229; PMCID: PMC7700057.

Smith CC, Bernstein LI, Davis RB, Rind DM, Shmerling RH. Screening for statin-related toxicity: the yield of transaminase and creatine kinase measurements in a primary care setting. Arch Intern Med. 2003 Mar 24;163(6):688-92. doi: 10.1001/archinte.163.6.688. PMID: 12639201.

Smith DK, Lennon RP, Carlsgaard PB. Managing Hypertension Using Combination Therapy. Am Fam Physician. 2020 Mar 15;101(6):341-349. PMID: 32163253.

Sofi F, Cesari F, Abbate R, Gensini GF, Casini A. Adherence to Mediterranean diet and health status: meta-analysis. BMJ. 2008 Sep 11;337:a1344. doi: 10.1136/bmj.a1344. PMID: 18786971; PMCID: PMC2533524.

Stamatakis E, Ahmadi MN, Friedenreich CM, et al. Vigorous Intermittent Lifestyle Physical Activity and Cancer Incidence Among Nonexercising Adults: The UK Biobank Accelerometry Study. JAMA Oncol. 2023;9(9):1255–1259. doi:10.1001/jamaoncol.2023.1830

Stead LF, Buitrago D, Preciado N, Sanchez G, Hartmann-Boyce J, Lancaster T. Physician advice for smoking cessation. Cochrane Database Syst Rev. 2013 May 31;2013(5):CD000165. doi: 10.1002/14651858.CD000165.pub4. PMID: 23728631; PMCID: PMC7064045.

Tessier, AJ., Wang, F., Korat, A.A. et al. Optimal dietary patterns for healthy aging. Nat Med (2025). https://doi.org/10.1038/s41591-025-03570-5

Toledo E, Salas-Salvadó J, Donat-Vargas C, Buil-Cosiales P, Estruch R, Ros E, Corella D, Fitó M, Hu FB, Arós F, Gómez-Gracia E, Romaguera D, Ortega-Calvo M, Serra-Majem L, Pintó X, Schröder H, Basora J, Sorlí JV, Bulló M, Serra-Mir M, Martínez-González MA. Mediterranean Diet and Invasive Breast Cancer Risk Among Women at High Cardiovascular Risk in the PREDIMED Trial: A Randomized Clinical Trial. JAMA Intern Med. 2015 Nov;175(11):1752-1760. doi: 10.1001/jamainternmed.2015.4838. Erratum in: JAMA Intern Med. 2018 Dec 1;178(12):1731-1732. doi: 10.1001/jamainternmed.2018.6460. PMID: 26365989.

Tran KB, Lang JJ, Compton K, et al The global burden of cancer attributable to risk factors, 2010–19: a systematic analysis for the Global Burden of Disease Study 2019 Lancet. 2022;400:563.

UKPDS Group, Effect of intensive blood-glucose control with metformin on complications in overweight patients with type 2 diabetes (UKPDS 34). UK

Prospective Diabetes Study (UKPDS) Group. Lancet. 1998 Sep 12;352(9131):854-65. Erratum in: Lancet 1998 Nov 7;352(9139):1558. PMID: 9742977.

University of Wisconsin Population Health Institute. County health rankings key findings 2018. http://www.countyhealthrankings.org/explore-health-rankings/rankings-reports/2018-county-health-rankings-key-findings-report. Accessed September 12, 2018.

University of Connecticut Rudd Center for Food Policy and Obesity. Increasing disparities in unhealthy food advertising targeted to Hispanic and black youth. http://uconnruddcenter.org/files/Pdfs/TargetedMarketingReport2019.pdf. Accessed January 19, 2019.

US Department of Agriculture, Economic Research Service. Interactive charts and highlights. 2018. https://www.ers.usda.gov/topics/food-nutrition-assistance/food-security-in-the-us/interactive-charts-and-highlights/. Accessed September 12, 2018.

USAFacts, https://usafacts.org/articles/obesity-rate-nearly-triples-united-states-over-last-50-years/ accessed on 07/06/2025

US Preventive Services Task Force; Krist AH, Davidson KW, Mangione CM, Barry MJ, Cabana M, Caughey AB, Davis EM, Donahue KE, Doubeni CA, Kubik M, Landefeld CS, Li L, Ogedegbe G, Owens DK, Pbert L, Silverstein M, Stevermer J, Tseng CW, Wong JB. Screening for Lung Cancer: US Preventive Services Task Force Recommendation Statement. JAMA. 2021 Mar 9;325(10):962-970. doi: 10.1001/jama.2021.1117. PMID: 33687470.

Vaughan AS, Coronado F, Casper M, Loustalot F, Wright JS. County-Level Trends in Hypertension-Related Cardiovascular Disease Mortality-United States, 2000 to 2019. J Am Heart Assoc. 2022 Apr 5;11(7):e024785. doi: 10.1161/JAHA.121.024785. Epub 2022 Mar 18. PMID: 35301870; PMCID: PMC9075476.

Virani SS, Alonso A, Benjamin EJ, Bittencourt MS, Callaway CW, Carson AP, Chamberlain AM, Chang AR, Cheng S, Delling FN, Djousse L, Elkind MSV,

Ferguson JF, Fornage M, Khan SS, Kissela BM, Knutson KL, Kwan TW, Lackland DT, Lewis TT, Lichtman JH, Longenecker CT, Loop MS, Lutsey PL, Martin SS, Matsushita K, Moran AE, Mussolino ME, Perak AM, Rosamond WD, Roth GA, Sampson UKA, Satou GM, Schroeder EB, Shah SH, Shay CM, Spartano NL, Stokes A, Tirschwell DL, VanWagner LB, Tsao CW; American Heart Association Council on Epidemiology and Prevention Statistics Committee and Stroke Statistics Subcommittee. Heart Disease and Stroke Statistics-2020 Update: A Report From the American Heart Association. Circulation. 2020 Mar 3;141(9):e139-e596. doi: 10.1161/CIR.0000000000000757. Epub 2020 Jan 29. PMID: 31992061.

Vittone, J., Gill, D., Goldsmith, A. et al. A multi-cancer early detection blood test using machine learning detects early-stage cancers lacking USPSTF-recommended screening. npj Precis. Onc. 8, 91 (2024). https://doi.org/10.1038/s41698-024-00568-z

Wickramaratne PJ, Yangchen T, Lepow L, Patra BG, Glicksburg B, Talati A, Adekkanattu P, Ryu E, Biernacka JM, Charney A, Mann JJ, Pathak J, Olfson M, Weissman MM. Social connectedness as a determinant of mental health: A scoping review. PLoS One. 2022 Oct 13;17(10):e0275004. doi: 10.1371/journal.pone.0275004. Erratum in: PLoS One. 2024 Nov 15;19(11):e0314220. doi: 10.1371/journal.pone.0314220. PMID: 36228007; PMCID: PMC9560615.

World Health Organization, Global immunization efforts have saved at least 154 million lives over the past 50 years, Joint News Release accessed on 05/12/2025 at https://www.who.int/news/item/24-04-2024-global-immunization-efforts-have-saved-at-least-154-million-lives-over-the-past-50-years

World Health Organization, Global Health Estimates: Leading Causes of Death accessed on 04/27/2025 at https://www.who.int/data/gho/data/themes/mortality-and-global-health-estimates/ghe-leading-causes-of-death

Wald DS, Law M, Morris JK, Bestwick JP, Wald NJ. Combination therapy versus monotherapy in reducing blood pressure: meta-analysis on 11,000 participants from 42 trials. Am J Med. 2009 Mar;122(3):290-300. doi: 10.1016/j.amjmed.2008.09.038. PMID: 19272490.

Wang L, Chen Z, Liu X, Wang L, Zhou Y, Huang J, Liu Z, Lin D, Liu L. GLP-1 Receptor Agonist Improves Mitochondrial Energy Status and Attenuates Nephrotoxicity In Vivo and In Vitro. Metabolites. 2023 Nov 1;13(11):1121. doi: 10.3390/metabo13111121. PMID: 37999218; PMCID: PMC10672795.

Wang L, Xu R, Kaelber DC, Berger NA. Glucagon-Like Peptide 1 Receptor Agonists and 13 Obesity-Associated Cancers in Patients With Type 2 Diabetes. JAMA Netw Open. 2024;7(7):e2421305. doi:10.1001/jamanetworkopen.2024.21305

Wang, SF., Tseng, LM. & Lee, HC. Role of mitochondrial alterations in human cancer progression and cancer immunity. J Biomed Sci 30, 61 (2023). https://doi.org/10.1186/s12929-023-00956-w

Weeldreyer NR, De Guzman JC, Paterson C, Allen JD, Gaesser GA, Angadi SS. Cardiorespiratory fitness, body mass index and mortality: a systematic review and meta-analysis. Br J Sports Med. 2025 Feb 20;59(5):339-346. doi: 10.1136/bjsports-2024-108748. PMID: 39537313; PMCID: PMC11874340.

Wei J, Galaviz KI, Kowalski AJ, Magee MJ, Haw JS, Narayan KMV, Ali MK. Comparison of Cardiovascular Events Among Users of Different Classes of Antihypertension Medications: A Systematic Review and Network Meta-analysis. JAMA Netw Open. 2020 Feb 5;3(2):e1921618. doi: 10.1001/jamanetworkopen.2019.21618. PMID: 32083689; PMCID: PMC7043193.

Xi B, Veeranki SP, Zhao M, Ma C, Yan Y, Mi J. Relationship of Alcohol Consumption to All-Cause, Cardiovascular, and Cancer-Related Mortality in U.S. Adults. J Am Coll Cardiol. 2017 Aug 22;70(8):913-922. doi: 10.1016/j.jacc.2017.06.054. Erratum in: J Am Coll Cardiol. 2017 Sep 19;70(12):1542. doi: 10.1016/j.jacc.2017.08.008. PMID: 28818200.

Yang E, Schutte AE, Stergiou G, Wyss FS, Commodore-Mensah Y, Odili A, Kronish I, Lee HY, Shimbo D. Cuffless Blood Pressure Measurement Devices-International Perspectives on Accuracy and Clinical Use: A Narrative Review. JAMA Cardiol. 2025 Apr 23. doi: 10.1001/jamacardio.2025.0662. Epub ahead of print. PMID: 40266607.

Yang S, Zhou Z, Miao H, Zhang Y. Effect of weight loss on blood pressure changes in overweight patients: A systematic review and meta-analysis. J Clin Hypertens (Greenwich). 2023 May;25(5):404-415. doi: 10.1111/jch.14661. Epub 2023 May 4. PMID: 37141231; PMCID: PMC10184479.

Yao H, Zhang A, Li D, Wu Y, Wang C, Wan J et al. Comparative effectiveness of GLP-1 receptor agonists on glycaemic control, body weight, and lipid profile for type 2 diabetes: systematic review and network meta-analysis BMJ 2024; 384 :e076410 doi:10.1136/bmj-2023-076410

Yedlapati SH, Khan SU, Talluri S, Lone AN, Khan MZ, Khan MS, Navar AM, Gulati M, Johnson H, Baum S, Michos ED. Effects of Influenza Vaccine on Mortality and Cardiovascular Outcomes in Patients With Cardiovascular Disease: A Systematic Review and Meta-Analysis. J Am Heart Assoc. 2021 Mar 16;10(6):e019636. doi: 10.1161/JAHA.120.019636. Epub 2021 Mar 13. PMID: 33719496; PMCID: PMC8174205.

Zhang H, Plutzky J, Skentzos S, Morrison F, Mar P, Shubina M, Turchin A. Discontinuation of statins in routine care settings: a cohort study. Ann Intern Med. 2013 Apr 2;158(7):526-34. doi: 10.7326/0003-4819-158-7-201304020-00004. PMID: 23546564; PMCID: PMC3692286.

Zhang WB, Milman S. Looking at IGF-1 through the hourglass. Aging (Albany, NY). 2022 Aug 25;14(16):6379-6380. doi: 10.18632/aging.204257. Epub 2022 Aug 25. PMID: 36063137; PMCID: PMC9467390.

Zhou D, Xi B, Zhao M, Wang L, Veeranki SP. Uncontrolled hypertension increases risk of all-cause and cardiovascular disease mortality in US adults: the NHANES III Linked Mortality Study. Sci Rep. 2018 Jun 20;8(1):9418. doi: 10.1038/s41598-018-27377-2. PMID: 29925884; PMCID: PMC6010458.

Zhou F, Jatlaoui TC, Leidner AJ, Carter RJ, Dong X, Santoli JM, Stokley S, Daskalakis DC, Peacock G. Health and Economic Benefits of Routine Childhood Immunizations in the Era of the Vaccines for Children Program - United States, 1994-2023. MMWR Morb Mortal Wkly Rep. 2024 Aug 8;73(31):682-685. doi:10.15585/mmwr.mm7331a2. PMID: 39116024; PMCID: PMC11309373.

www.ingramcontent.com/pod-product-compliance
Lightning Source LLC
Chambersburg PA
CBHW070620030426
42337CB00020B/3869